Psychedelic Information Theory

Shamanism in the Age of Reason

by James L. Kent

PIT Press
Supermassive, LLC
1122 E. Pike St. #679
Seattle, WA 98122

Copyright © 2010 by James L. Kent

Some rights reserved. Do not reproduce or reprint any section of this text without express permission from the author.

Library of Congress Publication Data

Kent, James L.

Psychedelic Information Theory: Shamanism in the Age of Reason / James L. Kent. First Edition.

Includes bibliographical references

ISBN 1453760172

EAN-13 9781453760178

http://psychedelic-information-theory.com

Keywords: Psychedelics, Entheogens, Hallucinogens, Consciousness, Perception, Pharmacology, Epistemology, Hallucination, Psychosis, Dreaming, Shamanism, Novelty Theory, Creativity, Nonlinear Dynamics, Chaos Theory

Psychedelic Information Theory

Shamanism in the Age of Reason

by James L. Kent

First Edition, PIT Press / Supermassive, LLC, 2010

For color images, updates, and links to references online:

http://psychedelic-information-theory.com

Images and Plates

01. Fractals generated by nature and computers — 08
02. Entopic patterns in phosphenes and prehistoric art — 10
03. Chaos stars, symbols of chaos magic — 13
04. Feedback circuits in visual perception — 28
05. Troxler's fading illusion — 39
06. Peripheral drift illusion — 41
07. Kalachakra time-wheels, mandalas, and calendars — 44
08. Stabilized and destabilized perception — 48
09. ADSR Envelope — 52
10. ADSR Envelope for N_2O and *Saliva divinorum* — 53
11. Molecular structure of glutamate and GABA — 57
12. Molecular structure of amines and hallucinogens — 58
13. Layers of the neocortex — 66
14. Biophillic fractals selected for intrinsic natural beauty — 76
15. Video feedback loop spinning towards central attractor — 77
16. Retino-cortical coupling pathways and mapping planes — 80
17. Entopic geometric form constants — 81
18. Examples of programmatic cellular automata — 83
19. Muscles of the eye — 85
20. Alien hallucination in entopic grid — 91
21. Molecular structure of acetylcholine and choline — 92
22. Hobson's AIM model — 93
23. Kitaoka's "Rotating Snakes" peripheral drift illusion — 98
24. Spiral and tunnel attractors in video feedback — 101
25. "Mushroom Inside" trance festival flyer — 112
26. Traditional shamen and medicine drums — 114
27. Shipibo textile patterns — 133
28. Hilbert plane-filling or Peano curves — 135
29. EEG bands over one level of activity — 142
30. Period doubling bifurcations in the logistics map — 176
31. Chladni figures created by standing interference patterns — 202

Preface

Psychedelic Information Theory (PIT) is a formal deconstruction of psychedelic hallucination, expanded consciousness, and shamanism, and as such it attempts to move topics which have traditionally been classified as metaphysics into fields of physics and mathematics. The goal of PIT is to unify all existing psychedelic research into a formal model which accurately describes the complex dynamics generated when a psychedelic drug is introduced into human neural and social networks. PIT is a general model which links psychedelic pharmacology directly to the nonlinear dynamics of expanded consciousness, neuroplasticity, shamanic technique, and tribal organization. This book should be equally enlightening for shamen, physicians, scientists, mathematicians, mystics, and anyone seeking to model or understand the functional limits of expanded consciousness.

PIT is presented as an introductory textbook for people with broad interests in consciousness, perception, psychedelics, hallucination, shamanism, dreaming, pharmacology, neuroplasticity, chaos theory, and related fields. Because PIT is meant to be an overview of a general theory which encompasses many diverse fields, it only scratches the surface of what could be a far larger and more detailed text. Students interested in further exploration on these topics should consult the bibliography and references for more avenues of research and discovery. For readers who are less scientifically inclined, or who seek a quick overview of the concepts covered in this text, an informal discussion of topics has been included in the appendixes. This discussion provides a brief summary of PIT and answers some of the most common questions raised in reaction to the text.

Sincerely,

James L. Kent

Table of Contents

Part I: Psychedelic Information Theory

01. What is Psychedelic Information Theory?	11
02. The Value of Psychedelic Information	15
03. Psychedelic Information Theory	21
04. What is Consciousness?	29
05. Limits of Human Perception	37
06. The Control Interrupt Model of Psychedelic Action	49
07. Psychedelic Pharmacology	57
08. $5\text{-}HT_{2A}$ Agonism and Multisensory Binding	67
09. What is Nonlinear Hallucination?	75
10. Entopic Hallucination	81
11. Eidetic Hallucination	90
12. Erratic Hallucination	99
13. Psychedelic Neuroplasticity	105

Part II: Shamanism in the Age of Reason

14. What is Shamanism?	115
15. An Overview of Physical Shamanism	120
16. Physical Shamanism and Shamanic Therapy	130
17. Hypnotic Entrainment and Induced Trance States	137
18. Psychic Bonding and Psi	143
19. Group Mind and Fluid Tribal Dynamics	148
20. Shamanic Sorcery	153
21. Spirits and Spiritual Communion	158
22. Information Genesis and Complexity	163

Appendixes

01. Conclusions and Discussion	170
02. Informal Discussion of Topics	179
03. About this Text	190
04. Bibliography and References	192
05. About the Author	203

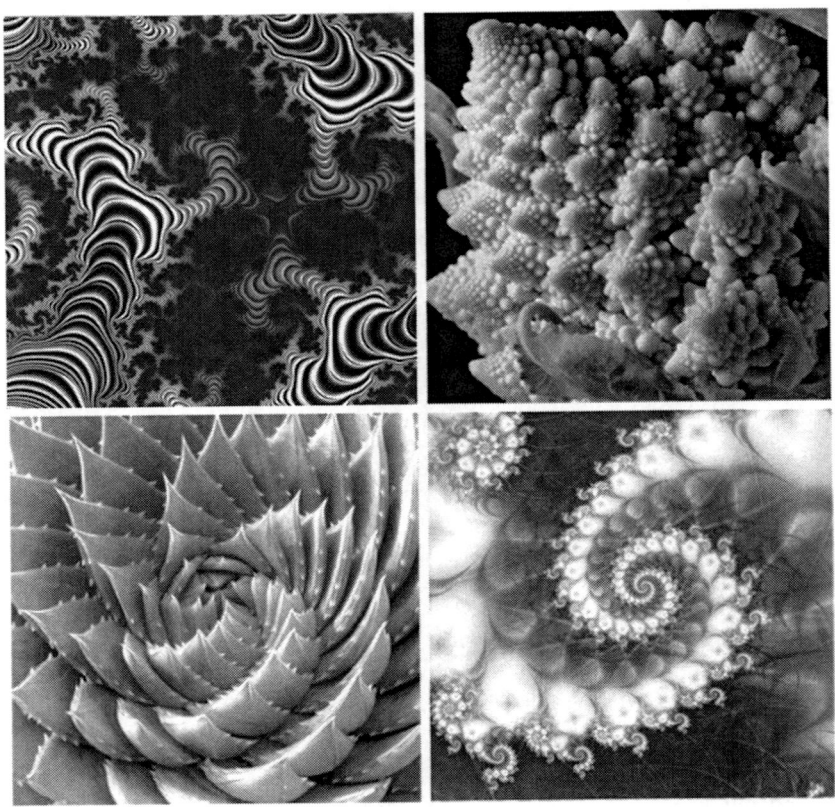

Figure 1. Fractals generated by computer programs and nature are examples of deterministic chaos in nonlinear systems, and share many formal similarities with psychedelic hallucinations. WikiMedia Commons.

Part I

Psychedelic Information Theory

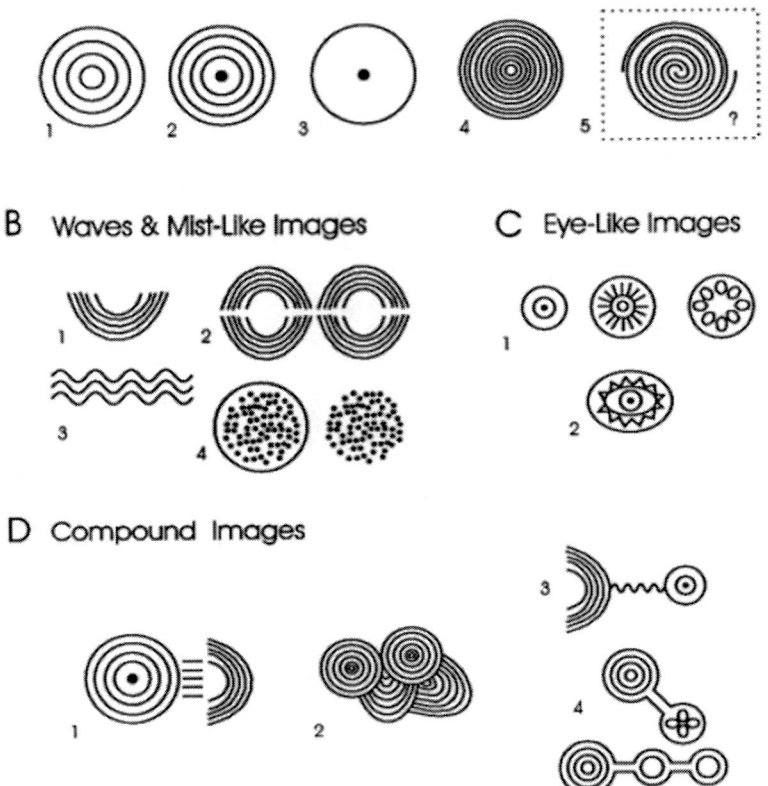

Figure 2. Images of internally generated sensations of light (phosphenes) with geometric shapes and no memory-based content, found in ethnographic reports and prehistoric rock art studies. From Nicholson and Firnhaber.

Chapter 01

What is Psychedelic Information Theory?

Psychedelic Information Theory (PIT) is the study of information creation in the human imagination, particularly in states of dreaming, psychosis, and hallucination. PIT seeks to model the functional output of human perception in order to extrapolate the limits and complexity of information arising in human altered states of consciousness.

The foundation of PIT lies in novelty theory, the study of increasing complexity of information over time. Novelty theory encompasses a large time-scale, but PIT is specifically focused on the spontaneous production of complex information in the human organism, which is also known as creativity theory or generative theory. Modeling the creation of information in the human brain requires formal definitions for perception, consciousness, and information, and as such PIT is also a work of systems theory, which posits that the potential output of any system can be fully described by the functional limitations of its components. PIT also draws on control theory, which models the stability and complexity of signal processing in dynamical systems. By applying control theory and systems theory to altered states of consciousness, PIT is an analysis of the nonlinear dynamics of hallucination and expanded states of consciousness. And finally PIT draws upon the fields of wave mechanics, neural oscillators, neuroplasticity, and the fundamentals of pharmacology, cognitive theory, and neural signaling as they apply to perception, memory, and consciousness; this also makes PIT a text on multidisciplinary neuroscience.

Why "Psychedelic" Information Theory?

The bulk of human consciousness exists in a linear range which goes from highly focused and alert to deep asleep and dreaming. Most states of consciousness are experienced uniformly and independently of each other along this linear spectrum. For instance, when you are asleep you are not awake; when you are focused you are not daydreaming; when you are anxious you are not relaxed. The fact that consciousness exists in only one state at one time is an indication that the system is linear and stable. When two distinct perceptions or states of consciousness overlap at the same time this is an indication that the system is unstable, and in most cases where divergent states of consciousness overlap the output is viewed as a pathology.[1] State-divergent pathologies are typically treated with drugs targeted to amplify the positive traits and/or dampen the negative traits.

The term psychedelic means "mind manifesting," which implies that all potential states of mind may be manifested under the influence of psychedelic drugs. If normal consciousness moves in a straight line along a spectrum of many possible states, psychedelics represent a unique and reversible destabilization of this linear spectrum where consciousness can assume multiple points of consciousness simultaneously. The most extreme divergent state of consciousness is described as being wide awake while simultaneously dreaming, a state clinically referred to as psychosis or hallucination. The emergence of multi-state consciousness under the influence of psychedelics represents a system that has destabilized from linear output and has become nonlinear and exponentially complex. Thus, in psychedelic perception the linear functions of consciousness diverge into a complex nonlinear state where multiple perspectives and analytical outputs may be experienced simultaneously.[2] According to PIT, this destabilized state of nonlinear complexity is where new information is generated in the human mind. Understanding the dynamics of this unique nonlinear function is essential to understanding the informational limits and potential complexity range of all human consciousness.

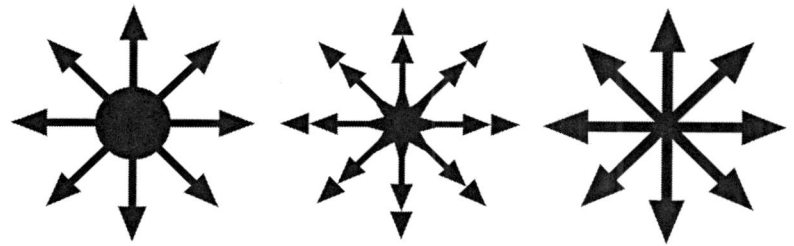

Figure 3. The eight-pointed star is a popular symbol of chaos magic. The arrows represent energy, or information, scattering at high velocity. This symbol is isomorphic of a nonlinear information system, like a universe, which starts at a single point and erupts outward in all directions.

What is "Shamanism in the Age of Reason"?

PIT seeks to describe a model of psychedelic activation that can be adapted to all possible permutations of human consciousness, including group mind states, mystical states, and transpersonal awareness. The ritual of using psychedelics to generate new information, bond with peer groups, and program human belief is traditionally called shamanism, so PIT is a study of the practice of shamanism, which can also be called applied psychedelic science. The practice of using ritual techniques of spiritual transcendence to manipulate belief systems has been popularly dubbed chaos magic, which is an occult blend of neo-shamanism, cognitive theory, and social theory (Fig. 3). Chaos and complexity are also popular terms applied to the study of nonlinear systems, such as fractals and cellular automata, making chaos magic and shamanism spirituo-scientific explorations of the generative function of nonlinear systems.

While PIT focuses on physiology over mythology, it is clear that there is a fundamental human desire to achieve states of consciousness subjectively described as Gnostic or spiritually enlightening. It is the conjecture of PIT that all mystical states, including healing and regenerative states, have unique formal nonlinear qualities that can be described in physical terms close enough to make good approximations. This means that PIT is also a work of technical shamanism, neuro-theology, or spiritual neuroscience, and can be referenced in the clinical application of psychedelic drugs in shamanic ceremony, mystical ritual, or psychedelic therapy.

Generic Application, Neutrality, Margin of Error

PIT does not attempt to provide precise definitions of consciousness, perception, or the psychedelic state. Instead PIT attempts to model an approximation of psychedelic consciousness based on the known functions and limits of human perception and cognition. According to PIT, if a functional reproduction of consciousness existed then it too could be made to have a psychedelic experience. This also makes PIT a text on artificial intelligence which can be tested in mechanical systems of perception. While this text may contain some assumptions and conjecture on human brain function, the fundamentals of PIT are generic enough to apply to any system of consciousness which relies on real-time frame perception for interacting with reality. Although the bulk of the text focuses on states of hallucinogenesis afforded most readily by the tryptamines LSD, psilocybin (magic mushrooms), and DMT (found in the South American brew ayahuasca), and their action at the 5-HT_{2A} receptor subtype, PIT strives to be generic and substance neutral, meaning that the fundamentals of PIT should apply to all drugs and techniques which produce hallucination, even though they may target different receptors and/or destabilize consciousness in a wholly unique way.

Notes and References

1. Some examples of pathologically divergent states of consciousness: Asleep and active is sleepwalking; excited and drowsy is narcolepsy; awake and rigid is Parkinson's Disease; awake and dreaming is psychosis; relaxed and nervous is anxiety disorder; fulfilled and sad is depressive disorder; and so on.

2. When a linear function diverges or bifurcates and begins plotting a range of multiple outputs for the same input, this can be called unstable, dynamic, nonlinear, complex, higher dimensional, undefined, and so on. It depends on how you model your system.

Chapter 02

The Value of Psychedelic Information

    A text called *Psychedelic Information Theory* raises the question, "What is Psychedelic Information, and why should we care?" Generally, psychedelic information is any information created in the mind of the subject during a psychedelic experience. Psychedelic information is generated spontaneously in reaction to the psychedelic catalyst; typically the subject has little or no control over the information generated in a psychedelic experience. Psychedelic information is almost always previously unknown to the subject and may appear to originate from an external source or materialize out of thin air. Psychedelic information typically takes the form of visual, audio, and sensory hallucination, but can also be abstract or gestalt like an emotional epiphany. Finally, psychedelic information applies to any art or concept that originates from or evokes psychedelic experience.
    This text focuses primarily on the physiological process underlying the spontaneous generation of psychedelic information, and how that information influences both personal and cultural identity. The fact that psychedelic information makes its way into popular culture is proof that humans find psychedelic information valuable, but it is still ambiguous if psychedelics add any real value to culture. Research has shown that spiders are affected by psychedelics,[1] as are rats,[2] cats,[3] monkeys,[4] and so on. However, there is little evidence that information other than noise is generated during psychedelic episodes in animals; the experience does not mean anything beyond a specific derangement of the senses. In contrast, the human adaptation to translate subjective experience into meaningful narrative is uniquely exploited by psychedelics. Psychedelics target perception, memory, and the complex emotions attached to symbols and concepts; the core functions humans

rely on to formulate belief. Because of this exploit, the result of the psychedelic catalyst in humans is the spontaneous generation of meaningful information which is imprinted into memory.

Any perceptual system can have a psychedelic experience,[5] but it takes abstract thinking and the interconnection between symbols, concepts, and emotions to make psychedelic information meaningful. Thus, the psychedelic experience does not create information in all systems of consciousness; the psychedelic experience only generates meaningful information in systems of consciousness with the capacity for abstract reasoning via symbolic logic and emotional attachment. Presumably any conscious system which emulates the functions of human abstract reasoning will also similarly generate meaningful information during a psychedelic experience.

The Value of Information

Within the set of information valuable to humans there are domains of descending importance. First there is information valuable to all organisms (biological information), then there is information valuable to all humans (species information), then there is information valuable only to a specific local group of humans (cultural information), and then there is information valuable only to a single human (personal information). All biological information and the most important bits of species information are genetic and are preserved through natural selection. Within the domain of human species importance there is also technological information (such as fire, tools, language, music, agriculture, science, etc.) which are culturally agnostic and serve the needs of the entire species equally. Technological information of species-level importance is equated with high value and will be adopted by all cultures over a short period. Species-level information has high durability and changes very slowly over time.

Cultural information falls in the category of language-based memes and regional or tribal traditions. Cultural information may be shared across cultures or may be restricted to a specific region or subculture. Cultural information is considered to be of medium value, low durability, and changes rapidly over time as the memes and traditions of culture change. Religion and artwork are examples of cultural information that typically only have value to their culture of origin, but occasionally ascend to species-level importance. Finally there is personal information, which is valuable only to a single individual. Personal information changes rapidly, is subject to experience and whim, and is only useful over the lifetime of the organism. Personal information has very low durability and low overall value.

The Value of Psychedelic Information

Psychedelic information is generated within the domain of the personal; yet many people who take psychedelics perceive the information as having species-level importance. There are a few reasons for this phenomena. The first, and easiest, is that psychedelics create states of mania and delusions of grandeur in which the subject feels that he or she is the most brilliant person on the planet, or that they are receiving supernatural prophecy. Secondly, the subject may experience archetypal visions or sensations of transcendence that are perceived to be of high religious or mystical importance. Thirdly, the subject may experience a deconstruction of consciousness associated with animal consciousness, reptilian consciousness, plant consciousness, the Gaian mind, genetic-level intelligence, or deep species memory; information perceived to be of value to all humans or all living creatures. Because psychedelics produce all of these experiences they are routinely perceived as having species-level importance.

Psychedelics are obviously useful in the domain of the personal; shamanism and psychedelic therapy rely on the information function of psychedelics to diagnose and heal. In the cultural domain psychedelics can be employed in ritual to build strong religious or tribal groups; they can be used in healing or sorcery; or they can be a catalyst for innovation and creative expression. Beyond this their value is ambiguous. There are some debates to be made in this area, such as pointing out that Francis Crick envisioned the spiral structure of DNA after he ingested LSD,[6] or that LSD helped Kary Mullis think up the PCR process that earned him a Nobel Prize in genetics.[7,8] To counter these arguments, both Crick and Mullis had been studying molecular biology for years trying to crack those very problems; LSD cannot take credit for anything more than helping Crick and Mullis organize their thoughts in a new way. We can point to great discoveries as examples of psychedelic information, but only a tiny fraction of all psychedelic information can claim this level of importance. Worse than this, erroneous psychedelic information claiming species-level importance has negative cultural value and dilutes the overall information marketplace, making psychedelic information almost statistically worthless.[9]

Probability dictates that most psychedelic information will have little or moderate value, and that the rare piece of psychedelic information will have extreme negative or positive value. It also follows that the more times a subject takes psychedelics the more likely it is they will generate information of high positive or negative value. Similarly, the more often a subject takes psychedelics the more likely they are to latch onto and subsequently reinforce information of high perceived value, either positive or negative. In this case the psychedelic becomes an information imprinting tool. In psychedelic imprinting the information is always subjectively perceived to be of high value, even if it is of low or even negative cultural value.[10]

Negative and Positive Information Value

It is easy to demonstrate that psychedelic information has value; cultures that use psychedelics as sacraments place high value on the information they receive; people will trade hard-earned cash for a psychedelic experience. But because the quality of psychedelic information has such a wide range it is easy to perceive psychedelics as having no value or, in the argument of prohibition, negative value. Psychedelic information with negative value can be described as that which is delusional, paranoid, false, or subverts the health of the individual or culture. Negative psychedelic experiences, or bummers, are a commonly reported element of psychedelic experimentation, but this does not necessarily make bummers negative. Some users claim that negative experiences have value because they provide emotional insight; others report that negative psychedelic experiences cause permanent psychological damage, which is extremely negative. In rare cases people act out and harm themselves or commit suicide on psychedelics. Obviously these are extreme examples of negative value, and these extreme examples are usually linked to mixing drugs, drug binging, or overdosing. There is an optimal dose range for any psychedelic substance; reports of negative effects increase once the optimal dose range is surpassed.[11]

Conversely, there is a range of psychedelic experience that is just as extreme but positive in value; the spiritual or therapeutic or entheogenic experience that adds value to the user and their culture. Having an extremely positive psychedelic experience does not happen by accident; there is nuance involved in selecting the proper dose, finding the right setting, and so on. By contrast, having a negative psychedelic experience is almost always an accident due to improper dose or setting. Therefore, the positive value of a psychedelic experience can be predicted and controlled up to a certain dose range, but beyond that the potential positive value drops and potential negative value increases.

Shamanism, which for the purposes of this text is defined as the practice of using psychedelics in ritual, employs specialized techniques to guide psychedelic information along desired pathways. Influencing and imprinting psychedelic information along positive pathways is perceived as spiritual, enlightening, and therapeutic; influencing or imprinting psychedelic information along negative pathways is perceived as mind control, black magic, or sorcery. Although the value of psychedelic information generated in any single episode is ambiguous, the practice of shamanism is a durable technology with species-wide application. Thus, shamanism is a technological subset of psychedelic information with high value to the entire species, even though the practice of shamanism can be employed to both positive or negative effect.

Notes and References

1. Christiansen A, Baum R, Witt P, "Changes In Spider Webs Brought About By Mescaline, Psilocybin And An Increase In Body Weight". JPET April 1962 vol.136 no.1 31-37.

2. Butters, Nelson, "The effect of LSD-25 on spatial and stimulus perseverative tendencies in rats". Psychopharmacology, Volume 8, Number 6 / November, 1966

3. Trulson M, Howell G, "Ontogeny of the behavioral effects of lysergic acid diethylamide in cats". Developmental Psychobiology Volume 17 Issue 4, Pages 329 - 346

4. Jarvik M, Chorover S, "Impairment by lysergic acid diethylamide of accuracy in performance of a delayed alternation test in monkeys". Psychopharmacology, Volume 1, Number 3 / May, 1960.

5. See Chapter 04, "What is Consciousness?".

6. Rees, Alun, "Nobel Prize genius Crick was high on LSD when he discovered the secret of life". Mail on Sunday, 8 August 2004.

7. Mullis, Kary, "Dancing Naked in the Mind Field". Vintage, NY, 2000.

8. Rabinow, Paul, "Making PCR: a story of biotechnology". University of Chicago Press, 1996.

9. The psychedelic community produces a new guru every decade or so, and the cultural contributions of these gurus trends from pseudo-scientific to outright fantastical. It is often difficult to tell if the contributions of psychedelic celebrities outweigh the more nonsensical memes they propagate.

10. Psychedelic imprinting can take many forms, and in some cases negative information can be imprinted into identity. Brainwashing is the act of imprinting another person against their will, which is viewed as negative. Self-brainwashing is the act of imprinting yourself with negative information either by choice or error. In self-brainwashing negative information typically assumes explicit paranoid or messianic themes. Extreme cases of psychedelic self-brainwashing will mimic elements of psychosis and persistent delusional disorder. See Chapter 13, "Psychedelic Neuroplasticity".

11. Hasler F, Grimberg U, Benz M, Huber T, Vollenweider F, "Acute psychological and physiological effects of psilocybin in healthy humans: a double-blind, placebo-controlled dose-effect study". Psychopharmacology, Volume 172, Number 2 / March, 2004.

Chapter 03

Psychedelic Information Theory

Like dreams, psychedelics are catalysts for generating information in the human imagination. There are many theories about the origin of this information: the subconscious; repressed emotions; the collective unconscious; genetic memory; spirit entities; alien transmission; junk data from neural excitation; and so on. Regardless of the origin it is widely accepted that psychedelics do generate information, and not merely junk data of questionable value. Psychedelics excel at producing salient information which can have a profound impact on the beliefs and identity of the subject.

The information generated by psychedelics is usually personal, but it can become transpersonal as psychedelic insights are shared with friends and the public. The rate of psychedelic information flow can be measured by the amount of explicit influence psychedelics have over any given culture, and the rate of flow is different for every culture. Some cultures repress anything resembling psychedelic information while others make it central to their spirituality.[1] Since the cultural revolution of the 1960s, psychedelic information flow has erupted into Western culture at an unprecedented rate. This rate of modern psychedelic information flow has had its ups and downs, but overall has remained relatively constant even in the face of global prohibition.[2]

The pathway of psychedelic information flow is simple and universally the same: 1) ingestion; 2) internal transmission; 3) internal integration; 4) cultural transmission; 5) cultural integration. Most psychedelic research focuses solely on internal transmission, the second stage of the psychedelic information process which is commonly called the trip. While the trip is certainly interesting it is still only one part of the larger overall process by which psychedelics influence both the individual and culture. Each part of this information process has its own patterns and predictable stages, and different portions of this text will attempt to illuminate one or more of these stages in the service of providing an overall understanding of how psychedelics impact culture. Below is a capsule summary of each stage in the psychedelic information process.

Ingestion

While it is difficult to define why people choose to take psychedelics, each society has its own rules which dictate who is allowed to ingest a psychedelic drug and in what context. In traditional settings ingestion is a spiritual exercise used to gain supernatural wisdom, and dosage is controlled ritually by the shaman. In modern Western culture the traditional rules have broken down and psychedelic ingestion has become complex and somewhat haphazard. In a modern context most people are introduced to psychedelics in mundane recreational circumstances, motivated by hedonism, curiosity, boredom, peer pressure, or rebellion. Sometimes an innate hunger for the mysterious drives ingestion. Typically the psychedelic user is seeking something, however vague that notion.

Internal Transmission

Internal transmission is where the psychedelic interacts with the neural network and new information is generated. Information in the psychedelic state is generated spontaneously within visual and audio hallucination; ideas which pop into the subject's imagination; novel juxtapositions of previous concepts; and removed perspectives that allow for new holistic analysis. This information can be literal or figurative; it can be abstract; it can come in words or phrases; it can be spoken or sung; it can be visual; it can emerge as epiphanies or brilliant ideas; it can be a recalled memory; it can be delivered by spirit entities in strange languages; and so on. The information density in a psychedelic session is layered, saturated, and colorfully detailed. Much of the information in a psychedelic hallucination may be accurately described as kaleidoscopic noise, but within this noise comes a wealth of salient content.[4]

In physical terms psychedelics create new information via spontaneous activation and organization of sensory and perceptual networks. Psychedelic information is experienced via direct neural firing and is transferred to memory via the creation and strengthening of synaptic connections in the neural network.[5] Psychedelic information generation takes energy, and the information processing capacities of the human brain are finite, and thus there is an upper limit to the amount of information that can be generated within a single psychedelic session before the brain begins to down-regulate in an attempt to return to baseline.[6]

Internal Integration

For many reasons there is loss of fidelity in the transmission of hallucinatory information from imagination into memory. Like a dream, memories of the psychedelic session must be compressed into manageable snippets that stand out within the larger wash of information. Although psychedelic hallucinations fade quickly they can have lasting emotional impact. How each person deals with the content of each experience is unique to their world view. Some people may choose to ignore content derived from the psychedelic experience; others may cherish anything they can remember and will scrutinize each vision in pursuit of higher metaphysical truth. During this process the information generated during the psychedelic trip is encoded into personal memory by forging and testing new synaptic pathways.

During post-psychedelic integration the subject may begin to re-assess and modify personal beliefs and behaviors. Cryptic and intense visions may be recalled over and over, or the subject may dwell obsessively on novel feelings experienced during their trip. The subject will typically review their psychedelic trip and create a lasting narrative of the journey, including what they experienced and what they learned. Integration is where the subject decides what happened in the experience. The content of the hallucination is not as important as the process by which the subject takes that content and shapes it into lasting memories, beliefs, and behaviors; this is the process of encoding psychedelic information into synaptic networks. Content generation without behavioral integration is essentially meaningless, so the true testament of psychedelic power is not the ability to produce visions, but the ability to imprint new information and transform belief.

Cultural Transmission

Psychedelic visions do not stay in the head; if they did there would be no psychedelic art, no psychedelic music, no psychedelic spirituality, and no psychedelic revolution. Psychedelics activate a process in which the realm of the psychological spills out into the realm of the physical. It is clear from 20th century history that psychedelics can fuel artistic expression, social experimentation, religious movements, and political activism. There is no other class of drugs which can claim to have such powerful cultural sway.[7] If psychedelics only produced hallucinations there would still be legitimate cause for fascination, but psychedelics also influence cultural movements, which makes them a global religious and political force to be reckoned with.

The ritual bonding of social groups though cultural transmission of psychedelic information is a subject that has been overlooked in almost all psychedelic research. Not only do psychedelics produce change at the individual level, they also produce changes at the group or tribal level, and thus they influence change in the social structures and goals of human culture. The spread of psychedelic information can be subtle or explicit, starting with the creation of art influenced by the psychedelic experience and culminating in the indoctrination of others into the psychedelic tribe through ritual sharing of the sacrament. Once a subject has been indoctrinated they too will spontaneously generate psychedelic information and begin sharing that information with others. This information process cascades from person to person until the cultural transmission of psychedelic memes reaches a tipping point and becomes openly adopted and even celebrated by the cultural mainstream.

Cultural Integration

By conservative estimates perhaps 10-15% of the population has ever tried a hallucinogen.[8] Despite such low levels of exposure the archetypes of psychedelic experience are well integrated into modern culture. Psychedelic subcultures (urban tribes) are active in every city on the planet. Annual psychedelic festivals, raves, and massives draw tens of thousands of people together from all continents.[9] Psychedelic influences appear constantly in modern fashion, music, visual arts, film, television, consumer products, marketing, packaging, advertising, videogames, and so on. Despite years of prohibition the promise of psychedelic spirituality and psychedelic therapy is still fresh in the public imagination.[10] The global cultural integration of psychedelic information may not be complete, but it is measurably on its way.

It has only been 50 years since the cultural revolution of the 1960s, and the speed with which psychedelics have influenced global culture is impressive. Over the decades the use of psychedelics has jumped generations, and each new generation rediscovers and repurposes the psychedelic ritual for its own needs. There are religious and political forces actively seeking to control or stop the use of psychedelics, but if current trends continue the complete cultural integration of psychedelic information seems inevitable. There may soon come a time when the global majority is in the psychedelic tribe, with the uninitiated minority self-excluded from the ritual. When psychedelic indoctrination reaches a majority of any population then that culture can be described as being saturated with psychedelic information. A culture that has become saturated with psychedelic information will naturally recognize psychedelic ritual as a legitimate rite of passage or spiritual practice.[11]

Psychedelic Information Process

The psychedelic information process is an observable phenomenon that has influenced cultures throughout history and is now affecting modern global culture. At the center of this information process is the pharmacological action of a small number of molecules hitting a tiny subset of neural receptors for a relatively short duration of time. The ongoing information process generated by this small pharmacological interaction goes far beyond the normal range of what we expect drugs to accomplish. Because psychedelics defy pharmacological rationality they are misunderstood, feared, and revered as spiritual in origin. This misunderstanding drives the psychedelic information process into divergent streams of theory and mythology, creating the tapestry of psychedelic propaganda, confusion, and disinformation we have today.

The divergence of psychedelic information and existence of competing schools of psychedelic ideology demonstrates there is no one objective and true psychedelic ideology; any ideology can be influenced and amplified by the psychedelic information process. The psychedelic information process is neutral and ideology non-specific; it applies equally to learning, creativity, mind-control, brainwashing, mysticism, sorcery, and healing. The psychedelic process and psychedelic archetypes can be co-opted by any religious or political group for personal power gain, and psychedelics can be used as weapons as easily as they can be used as medicines or sacraments.[12] The only constant between all divergent schools of psychedelic ideology is the physical process that stimulates the flow of novel information through human neural networks. The study of this information process is known as Psychedelic Information Theory.

Notes and References

1. Psychedelic information flow within any culture is a function of religion and politics. Traditional shamanic cultures value psychedelic information as a ritual form of bonding, healing, and discovery, and encourage psychedelic information flow. Industrialized cultures with centralized beliefs view psychedelic information as subversive and anti-authoritarian, and repress psychedelic experimentation out of fear of losing centralized control.

2. A close scrutiny of late 20th century history indicates that there was a small decline in psychedelic interest in the late 1970s and 1980s, followed by a global resurgence of underground psychedelic interest in the 1990s, and a complete return to psychedelic research at the turn of the 21st century. Prohibition may slow the flow of psychedelic information, but it does not stop it.

4. The content of psychedelic hallucinations has been described vividly in many places. See "Tripping" by Charles Hayes, or the Erowid.org Experience Vaults for hundreds of fascinating first person accounts.

5. See Chapter 13, "Psychedelic Neuroplasticity".

6. Gresch PJ, Smith RL, Barrett RJ, Sanders-Bush E., "Behavioral tolerance to lysergic acid diethylamide is associated with reduced serotonin-2A receptor signaling in rat cortex". Neuropsychopharmacology. 2005 Sep;30(9):1693-702.

7. Since psychoactive drugs shape politics and warfare around the world, the claim that psychedelics are more influential on culture and cultural movements than other drugs can be easily disputed. However, psychedelics are unique in their ability to quickly catalyze tribal subcultures bent on spontaneous altruism, populist activism, and free radicalism.

8. HHS/SAMHSA, Office of Applied Studies, "Ecstasy, Other Club Drugs, & Other Hallucinogens". Internet Reference, 2008.

9. Modern psychedelic festivals can be traced to the "Be-ins" and "Acid Tests" of San Francisco in the late 1960s, made famous by Tom Wolfe's "The Electric Kool-Aid Acid Test". These festivals evolved into Woodstock, the Grateful Dead circuit, the Rainbow Family, Rave culture, Burning Man, the Boom Festival, the Love Parade, and other gatherings around the world dedicated to psychedelic music, art, and culture. Attendance at the largest of these annual festivals is regularly in the tens to hundreds of thousands of people.

10. The 2006 psilocybin and mysticism study by Roland Griffiths brought new enthusiasm to mixing psychedelic spirituality with clinical therapy.

11. It is easy to claim that traditional tribal societies are saturated with psychedelic information, but modern society is not far behind. Western media is filled with psychedelic imagery and fascinated by altered states. In the United States, ayahuasca and peyote are already recognized as legitimate religious sacraments within specific churches, and psychedelic drug experimentation is a common rite of passage among university students.

12. Groups linked to the weaponized use of psychedelics include the Manson Family, the SLA, Aum Shinrikyo, the CIA, and the United States Department of Defense.

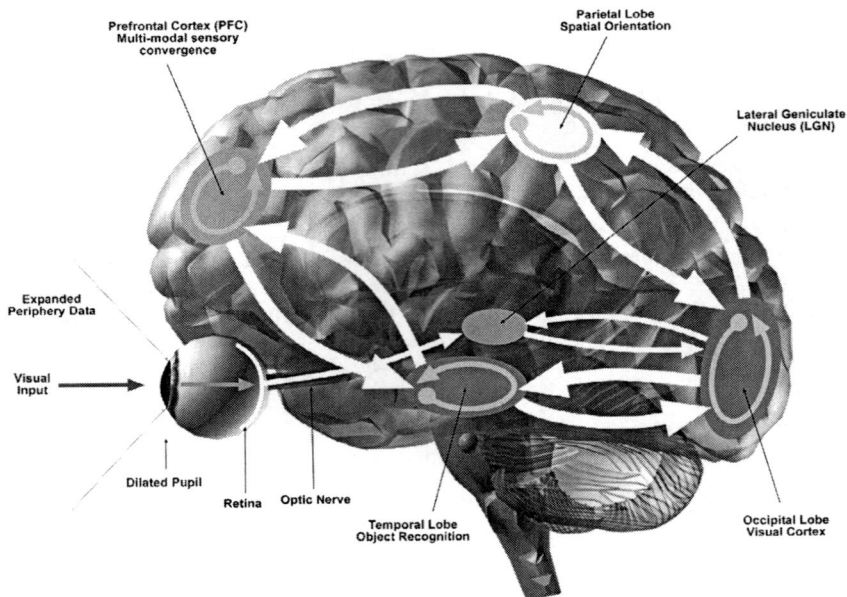

Figure 4. Feedback circuits in visual perception pathways. Sensory signal in human consciousness projects up and around the brain like a wave as consciousness arises in distinct stages. Sensation begins with the sensory organs and feeds into the thalamus (through the LGN for visual pathways), which filters and routes sensation into higher areas of the cortex. Recognition happens quickly and instinctively in the thalamus and medial temporal lobe, focusing attention on salient information. Memory identifies incoming signal moving upward in the cortex, passing data through parallel layers of spatial and object recognition along dorsal and ventral pathways. Multisensory perception finally converges in the pre-frontal cortex as a parsed reconstruction of reality is presented for informing real-time behaviors.

Chapter 04

What is Consciousness?

Since this text is about the manipulation of consciousness it is beneficial to have working definition for this term. Consciousness is defined here as a dynamical information processing system with specific functions and emergent operating properties, all of which are necessary to maintain system stability.[1] The minimum specific functions for any conscious system are: 1) perception 2) recognition 3) memory 4) recall, and 5) behavior. The minimum specific operating properties for any conscious system are: 1) modular coherence 2) linear stability 3) feedback control 4) adaptability, and 5) self-awareness. When all of these functions and operating properties are working in tandem you get something resembling human consciousness.[2] When one or more of the five essential functions is degraded then consciousness slides into semi-conscious, subconscious, or unconscious modes. When one or more of the five operating properties is degraded then consciousness becomes unstable and loses fidelity. A description of the functions and operating properties of consciousness follows.

Five Basic Functions of Consciousness

All conscious systems rely on five basic functions to interact with the environment in real time.

Perception

A conscious system must receive input, this input is called perception. For humans, perceptual input is received as sense data moving towards the brain from the peripheral nervous system. Sensation does not become actual perception until it is routed up through the thalamus and into higher cortical areas for processing. Humans also perceive internal thoughts and feelings, their own external behaviors, and small pieces of their dreams. Perception is linear, it feeds back on itself through behavior and recall, and its primary function is to observe changes in environment over time. Errors in human perception are sometimes called hallucination.

Recognition

Data from perception is parsed and matched against known salient patterns; this process is called recognition. Human recognition is driven by hormonal reaction to salient patterns; patterns which have high emotional resonance. Human recognition utilizes fast nonlinear analysis over slow semantic analysis. Fast recognition has high utility but low fidelity, meaning it works quickly but must be double-checked by linear memory for accuracy. Recognition is contextual, multisensory, associative, and its function is to find salient data in incoming perception. Nonlinear recognition errors include false identification, misrepresentation, and déjà vu.

Memory

All salient patterns are stored in memory. Patterns stored in memory are matched against incoming data for recognition; they are also matched against possible solutions for recall. In humans memory is imprinted by emotional resonance, reinforced through linear repetition, and potentiated though nonlinear contextual association. Human memory has many layers; semantic, eidetic, associative, and potentially holographic. Multi-layered human memory involves long-term potentiation and lossy compression, but this compression also includes indexing redundancy to serve fast recall and recognition of salient data.

Recall

Recall uses associative patterns stored in memory to make informed decisions based on logic. Unlike recognition, which is spontaneous and intuitive, recall uses negative feedback to inhibit detrimental solutions and positive feedback to stimulate advantageous solutions. Recall is cyclical and associative, meaning it can use both negative and positive feedback to cycle through and evaluate many hypothetical scenarios before resting on a final decision.[3] The main function of recall is to analyze patterns stored in memory to inform intelligent decisions and behaviors in real time.

Behavior

A conscious system performs behaviors based on input. Human behavior takes the form of both internal and external actions. Internal behaviors, such as thinking thoughts and feeling emotions, transform memory and recall into logical decisions; external behaviors translate internal decisions into outward actions. Human behavior is linear and serial; behaviors are performed in sequence one at a time, typically with thoughts and emotions preceding and informing the intent of action. Both internal and external behaviors feed back into perception, closing the loop on the perceptual feedback process.

Operating Properties of Consciousness

When all of the functions of consciousness are up and running the system begins to take on certain familiar operating properties. These basic properties are what we would expect from any conscious system, and any conscious system that loses these properties will also become unstable and lose fidelity of perception and memory.

Modular Coherence

In order to perform like a seamless, integrated system, consciousness must have some means of synchronizing performance between modular sub-functions. Functional cooperation between different areas of the brain is measured in terms of coupled neural oscillators, neural spike synchrony, and coherence of network oscillations.[4] Waking consciousness oscillates within the alpha and beta ranges; high frequency gamma coherence is associated with the fast binding of cortical networks necessary for perception and consciousness.[5] Modular coherence is the first operating property of a conscious system; precise timing between all areas is necessary for multisensory integration. Without coherence the modular sub-functions of consciousness lose interoperability and destabilize.

Linear Stability

Consciousness can perform many different functions, but it only performs one function at a time. The functional range of consciousness is linear and moves predictably from state to state with the passage of time. Consciousness transitions seamlessly from one behavior to the next. Consciousness retains state data and reacts logically to environmental change. In conscious systems the perception of the passage of time remains constant. The ability to remain focused on the environment and perform sequenced, goal-oriented behaviors in real-time is an operational baseline for all conscious systems.

Feedback Control

Conscious systems must be able to monitor and control their own stability and perform behaviors to modulate system input and output. All conscious systems must have some form of feedback control to retain object focus, retain state data, refine behaviors, perform state transitions, and maintain linear stability. Without feedback control, a dynamical information processing system is prone to output exuberance, memory overload, and error.[6]

Adaptability

A conscious system must be able to store patterns, predict outcomes, learn new behaviors, and react to external variable change. Adaptability and the ability to learn from experience is an epiphenomena or spontaneous operating property of a functionally stable consciousness. Intelligent systems that do not exhibit adaptability only mimic some of the functions and properties of consciousness without actually achieving full consciousness.

Self-Awareness

A conscious system must be aware of itself and be able to recognize other conscious systems. Self-awareness is an epiphenomena of the functions and properties of consciousness maintaining linear stability through time. Self-awareness and the ability to recognize and interact with other conscious systems may be the truest and most objective test of any stable consciousness.

Modular Consciousness

The most dramatic way to demonstrate the fragility of consciousness is to lose it. We sleep every night, and sleeping is a very limited form of consciousness where most of the functions and properties disappear. When we sleep we cannot hold state information from one moment to the next, thus we lose contextual data and self-awareness. In dreams we have perceptions and perform behaviors, but they are not linear nor do we have much control over them. In deep sleep all functions of consciousness go offline and almost entirely shut down. When we wake up these functions slowly return and then re-stabilize into an alert waking mode. Consciousness turns itself off; consciousness turns itself back on.

Sleeping and dreaming demonstrate that the basic functions of consciousness are modular and interdependent; they can operate individually as well as in specialized groupings. The modular functions of consciousness can be switched off and on in any order without affecting the long-term stability of the fully operational system. The modularity of consciousness becomes evident in cases of brain trauma or mental illnesses where the subject loses some functions of consciousness but retains others.[7] When consciousness is stable we cannot tell it is modular; it runs as a seamless whole or an integrated system. When consciousness destabilizes the modular units uncouple and reveal themselves to be sub-personal pieces of a larger identity process. The loss of multisensory perception and the splintering of consciousness into multiple independent processes can accurately be described as an altered state of consciousness.

Psychedelic Consciousness

If consciousness is modular and the modular functions can interoperate in multiple configurations, it is reasonable to assume there are multiple configurations of sub- and meta- consciousness that are rarely explored. The linear states of consciousness we experience daily are controlled by a top-down homeostatic regulator,[8] but when we short-circuit this regulator we find that modular sub-functions of consciousness can be destabilized, uncoupled, and accessed in novel ways. All forms of mysticism rely on radical destabilization of homeostasis.[9] EEG studies of subjects with hallucinogen persisting perception disorder (HPPD) have shown that when the visual cortex loses coherence with other areas of the brain and coherence among local visual networks increases, spontaneous hallucinations are produced.[10] Sensory deprivation for as little as fifteen minutes is all that is necessary to uncouple the visual cortex and have it start producing coherent self-sustaining hallucinations.[11] This can be described as sleep onset visualization, similar to daydreaming or lucid dreaming, and is sometimes called the prisoner's cinema because extended periods of solitary confinement also produce this effect, as does macular degeneration of the retina. This demonstrates that when modular functions of the brain are uncoupled from top-down coherence they do not always disappear, they may also spontaneously organize into more locally coherent configurations. This uncoupled and locally coherent activity can produce wandering or non-linear sensation in lower brain areas which floats up to conscious awareness as linear perception. This is a neat formal definition for states of dreaming, creative visualization, and hallucination.

Psychedelic Information Theory posits that the uncoupled sub-functions of modular consciousness, acting either alone or in novel peer groupings, are responsible for the subjective altered states classified as hallucinogenic, dissociative, and psychedelic. All hallucinogens must first destabilize top-down coherence of consciousness to produce novel states of spontaneous organization between the modular sub-units; this is how all hallucination begins. Dissociatives disrupt top-down coherence by blocking the excitatory pathways that allow the modular units to communicate. Psychedelics have a more subtle effect on top-down coherence; they periodically interrupt or excite the modulatory frequency of multisensory frame binding, causing perception to destabilize into energetic nonlinear configurations.[12] By destabilizing the top-down control of consciousness, psychedelics allow the modular sub-functions to wander and/or interact with coupled peers in dedicated subsystems; similar to the dedicated circuit created between perception and memory when dreaming.

Destabilizing or splintering consciousness into novel configurations is the essence of psychedelic exploration. When consciousness bifurcates or splits, subjective perception instantly becomes more chaotic and complex. Splintered consciousness may actually appear to be in two places at once, stuck in a superposition between waking and dreaming, finding stability in two simultaneous perceptual states, also know as multi-stability a multi-stable state. Novel configurations of splintered or multi-stable consciousness can be described as nonlinear, complex, meta, transpersonal, depersonalized, faceted, holistic, higher-dimensional, expanded, mystical, subconscious, semi-consciousness, and so on. Splintering, re-configuring, and rebuilding the modular sub-units of identity are techniques that may be applied in brainwashing or metaprogramming,[13] but also fall under the rubric of mysticism and shamanism. By subverting and re-organizing the modular functions of linear consciousness, psychedelics expand the functional range of consciousness to include many novel states of multi-stable complexity. These complex perceptual states, also known as expanded states of consciousness, are the origin of hallucination and the source of all the psychedelic information that has influenced human mythology, religion, art, science, and culture.

Notes and References

1. There is a popular school of thought which posits that consciousness precedes physicality, and that for there to be atoms and molecules and galaxies there must first be consciousness. This is a very broad definition of consciousness which should be saved for more metaphysical discussions.

2. The functions and operating properties of consciousness described here are a simplification of the functions of the human brain, but they are an ample enough description for modeling human consciousness in any environment.

3. This definition of deliberative recall is simplified and based on principles of deductive and inductive reasoning. This definition compresses a much larger discussion on the various types of neural logic and does not account for human emotional irrationality, but it is the minimum definition needed to model the output of human reasoning.

4. The so-called "binding problem" of multisensory perception is approached from a variety of directions, but current theories rely on measuring the strength, frequency, synchrony, and resonance of spike waves propagating through neural assemblies. There are many ways to estimate the relative cooperation between separated brain areas based on their wave properties. Coherence is a term used to indicate strong signal cooperation between

separated areas. Areas that are high in coherence may act like coupled oscillators in a feedback circuit, or they may take the form of parallel circuits engaged in a synchronized but distributed processing task.

5. Meador KJ, et al., "Gamma coherence and conscious perception". Neurology 2002;59:847-854.

6. WikiPedia.org, "Control Theory". Internet Reference, 2010.

7. The most compelling examples of mental illnesses which destabilize consciousness are Alzheimer's disease, which affects memory, and schizophrenia, which affects coherence and linear stability. These two examples compress a much larger discussion of how the degradation or loss of specific functions and operating properties of consciousness lead to specific pathologies.

8. Top-down modulation of waking consciousness is a function of aminergic modulation in the forebrain – serotonin and dopamine focusing and maintaining attention – but total homeostatic regulation of brain and body is generally considered to be a function of the hypothalamus. From WikiPedia: "The hypothalamus co-ordinates many hormonal and behavioral circadian rhythms, complex patterns of neuroendocrine outputs, complex homeostatic mechanisms, and many important behaviors."

9. Fasting, chanting, meditation, trance-dancing, isolation tanks, mind machines, and other non-drug visionary practices are rituals designed to destabilize homeostasis through deprivation and hypnotic repetition. Psychedelic drugs achieve more dramatic results by directly interrupting neuromodulatory pathways at the receptor site.

10. Abraham HD, Duffy FH, "EEG coherence in post-LSD visual hallucinations". Psychiatry Res. 2001 Oct 1;107(3):151-63.

11. Mason OJ, Brady F, "The psychotomimetic effects of short-term sensory deprivation". J Nerv Ment Dis. 2009 Oct;197(10):783-5.

12. See Chapter 06, "Control Interrupt Model of Psychedelic Action".

13. Metaprogramming is the term John Lilly chose in the text, "Programming and Metaprogramming in the Human Biocomputer". Splintering is a term used in brainwashing to describe the process of breaking the subject's identity into multiple pieces through stress exercises, making them vulnerable to imprinting and manipulation.

Chapter 05

Limits of Human Perception

Any discussion of psychedelic hallucination is a discussion of the spontaneous emergence of information in human perception. Human perception is limited by the capacity of sense organs; the speed and architecture of the neural network; and the number of distinct perceptions the brain can analyze at any one time. Despite functional limitations, human consciousness is seamless, meaning that each perception and behavior flows smoothly from one to the next. When consciousness is stable, perception and behavior is seamlessly integrated; when consciousness destabilizes, perception and behavior lose cohesion until we are no longer in control of our thoughts and actions. Destabilization of consciousness can happen all at once, in the case of being knocked unconscious, but more often it happens incrementally, as in going to sleep.

Psychedelics are unique in that they can both enhance and degrade perceptual limitations by orders of degrees; psychedelics can obscure and distort perceptual data, or they can enhance resolution and generate expanded states of consciousness. These contrasting results may be dose dependent, but it is also possible that psychedelics simultaneously produce perceptual degradation and enhancement. Psychedelic hallucinations are often described as being beyond the limits of human imagination, a trait which is offered as de-facto evidence of expanded consciousness or supernatural dominion. Since the boundaries of the human imagination can be modeled with some close degree of accuracy, any substantial discussion about the nature of psychedelic hallucination must therefore start with some basic assumptions about the limitations of human perception, and thus the functional limitations of expanded consciousness.

The Visual Spectrum

The human visual spectrum has evolved to work best in a small window of sunlight penetrating the Earth's atmosphere, comprising the white-light band seen in a rainbow; roughly the 400-790 THz (terahertz) energy range which oscillates on the order of hundreds of trillions of cycles per second. The smallest wavelength of visible light is violet, which is only 380 nm (nanometers) wide and travels with the highest frequency. Red, by contrast, is 750 nm long on the other end of the visible spectrum, and at twice the length it travels at half the frequency.[1] Unlike some organisms, the human eye does not see into ultraviolet or infrared rages, nor does it see microwaves, radio waves, x-rays, gamma rays, or anything that falls out of the visual spectrum. This also applies to night vision and dark-adapted vision. The dark-adapted eye utilizes the rod cells as opposed to the cone cells of daylight vision; rod cells are more photosensitive and more numerous, but they lack the color sensitivity and detail resolution of daylight rendering.[2]

Subjects on psychedelics often report increased luminosity and saturation of colors, as well as halos or auras of light surrounding objects; this implies an increase in color saturation and photosensitivity likely related to dilated pupils associated with $5-HT_{2A}$ agonism. In closed-eye or low-light environments subjects report vividly saturated geometric matrices rendered in swirling palettes of fluorescent purple and neon green.[3] All of these reports fall within the expected range of an overly saturated visible color spectrum, with the dark-adapted eye finding more sensitivity in the shorter-wavelength, higher-frequency, violet to green ranges.

There is speculation that psychedelic hallucination is the result of tuning the brain to receive cosmic radiation at a wider bandwidth than normal; bands associated with electromagnetic, metaphysical, morphogenetic, Akashic, or geomagnetic fields. This so-called spectral argument posits that instead of producing consciousness, the human brain acts as a radio receiver for consciousness, and psychedelics allow the user to tune the brain to new perceptual frequencies, possibly higher dimensional in nature. This metaphor may make intuitive sense, but no research exists to confirm any spectral advantage to psychedelics other than increased photosensitivity and some visual acuity at low doses.[4,5,6] Subjective reports indicate that psychedelics may increase auditory or synesthetic sensitivity to electromagnetic background noise, and the perception of energy fields or auras emanating from living organisms is reported often enough to warrant further scientific scrutiny, but these claims have not been tested rigorously enough to be conclusive.[7] The spectral argument is further weakened by the observation that if the human eye can be tuned to see a novel frequency range, a mechanical spectrum analyzer should also be able to pick up information on that same frequency. To date no hidden psychedelic spiritual energy fields have been detected by even the most sensitive spectral scanning devices.

Figure 5. Troxler's fading illusion demonstrates temporal decay of peripheral filling. Stare at the dot in center of image and hold eyes perfectly still for a count of 20. The border around the dot will being to fade. Blinking or moving the eyes will bring the fading areas back. From WikiPedia.

Visual Frame Aliasing

Seamless perception relies on rapid frame updating to render external changes in real time. Humans can render changes in reality at roughly 13-15 frames per second (fps, or Hz), which means that human reality fully refreshes roughly once every 77 milliseconds (ms), and open-eye saturation of peripheral filling fully fades at around 10-20 seconds (Fig. 5). Human frame perception is exploited by animation and film, which updates at 24 fps, and television, which updates near 30 fps. Computer monitors and high-definition televisions refresh at 60 Hz or higher, and at this rate human perception of motion is entirely seamless.[8] The rate of human frame perception corresponds roughly to the alert beta range of waking human consciousness (12-30 Hz) seen in EEG readings.[9] Any event which happens faster than $1/60^{th}$ of a second (16.6 ms) falls between perceptual frames and is considered to be subliminal or imperceptible to human consciousness.[10] Seamless frame rendering is also called temporal aliasing, and can be subverted by a variety of common phenomena, including stroboscopic lights which break motions into jerky snapshots, and wagon-wheel illusions where rotating spokes appear to stop or spin backwards.[11,12,13]

In addition to retaining visual information, perceptual frames hold the totality of multi sensory rendering. Smooth frame aliasing preserves semantic state information from one moment to the next, and retains fidelity of information held in working memory. There is evidence that the brain can track multiple object layers for each frame;[14] possibly corresponding to the number of distinct items we can sustain in working memory, which is about seven.[15] Frame rendering is a distributed cortical task modulated by the aminergic system. High aminergic modulation of the frontal lobe is a good indicator of external frame alertness. Any drug which interrupts the precise timing of the aminergic modulatory system will also disrupt the seamless nature of temporal frame aliasing in the same way that a strobe light disrupts the motion of a spinning wheel. Temporal aliasing hallucinations include frame stacking, frame delay, frame freezing, frame reverse, frame echo, and infinite frame regression; all of which are considered to be uniquely psychedelic.[16] The sensation of hallucinogenic frame stacking indicates that psychedelics may create a temporary frame decay buffer that allows for simultaneous multi-frame analysis and increased complexity of visual comprehension. Subverting or enhancing the limits of visual frame aliasing is an indication of expanded consciousness.

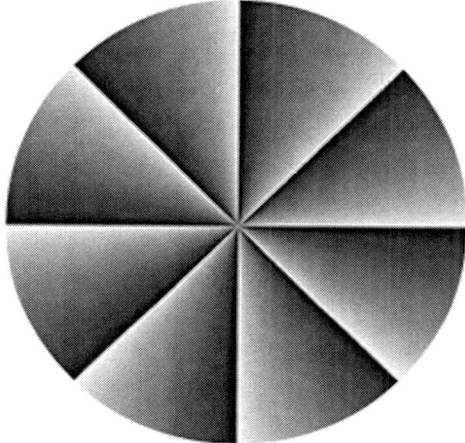

Figure 6. The peripheral drift illusion (PDI) is easily seen when this image is in the visual periphery. Research suggests the illusion is based on temporal differences in tracking luminance along four degrees of gradation. The four-step gradient processing produces a temporally mismatched contrast signal that fools the peripheral motion system. WikiPedia, Faubert & Herbert, 1998.

Visual Frame Resolution

Human visual resolution is limited by a number of factors. The first limitation is the density and distribution of retina in the eye; 130 million photoreceptors feeding into 1.2 million optic projections, with a spatial compression ratio of roughly 100 to 1. Photoreceptors in the eye are distributed in rings with color-sensitive cones clustering towards the center and contrast-sensitive rods filling the periphery.[17] Despite the large number of photoreceptors the field of vision is incomplete. Including the blind spot where the retina attaches to the optic nerve, as much as 20% of peripheral vision contains gaps that must be filled with progressive rendering. Incoming rings of visual data must be smoothed into lines and shades in the visual cortex; a process that can produce artifacts of the spatial network when destabilized.[18] The smoothed visual image is then passed forward in two divergent projections for spatial and object analysis, and the finished image reaches multi-modal convergence in the PFC (Fig. 4).[19] This is a fair bit of signal juggling for any processor to handle at 15 frames per second.

Even though human vision employs elaborate compression and reconstruction techniques, the human eye can detect visual detail at resolutions into the micrometer range. From a meter's distance the human eye cannot detect detail under 100 micrometers in length, making print resolutions of 300 dots-per-inch (DPI) entirely seamless. Some estimates put the detail of human visual resolution at 14 million pixels per the entire visual field; or by the 3D topographical field-rendering limit of 10 billion triangles per second, or 760 million triangles per frame.[8] Human detail resolution is only reliable near the center of vision; many optical illusions exploit perceptual filling functions of the periphery (Figs. 5 & 6).[20,21,22] Given the mechanical shortcomings of peripheral rendering, these estimates should be taken as visual saturation points as opposed to functional capacities.

The rendering of visual information may be the most complex and energy-intensive task of the human brain. Seamless visual perception requires precise neural firing. When perception destabilizes the visual field falls apart; the most commonly reported form of visual destabilization is diplopia or double-vision. Since visual rendering is so rich and complex, it is potentially the easiest part of the brain to destabilize. In other words, visual rendering is so elaborate and time-dependent it can be easily fooled by hallucination and illusion.

Dreaming, Imagination, Psychosis, Hallucination

While the information resolution of imagination and dreams is difficult to measure, it is widely agreed that dream perception is less resolved in detail than waking perception. Dreams are incomplete; contextual state data is not retained from frame to frame; and thus the durability of dream data falls apart under close scrutiny. Sometimes dreams can be vivid to the point of being indistinguishable from reality, containing people and places and narratives that retain state information over many different sequences, but more often dreams are fleeting and half remembered, lasting only a few seconds before fading.

Visual rendering of human imagination is more durable than dreams, but is also very low in resolution. Humans can imagine objects, people, and places in their minds, but human visual imagination is not typically photorealistic. Human memory is more semantic than eidetic, meaning that waking thoughts are mostly verbal, emotional, and only minimally visual. Most humans can imagine basic shapes, outlines, and sensual concepts; a smaller percentage can imagine topographical maps and rotate 3D objects in their mind. Visualizing a simple object like a cube or a pyramid is a cognitive task that requires full concentration; and even at peak visualization the internalized form rarely rises beyond a blurry silhouette. The exception to this limitation is dreaming or daydreaming, when eidetic or photographic snapshots bubble up into consciousness almost fully-formed. The emergence of dreamlike eidetic information into waking consciousness is usually a spontaneous reflex; few people have full control over photorealistic rendering of imagination and memory.[23,24]

Having fully-formed visions spontaneously erupting into consciousness is sometimes called overactive imagination, daydreaming, vivid memory recall, eidetic memory, photographic memory, emergent ideation, hallucination, or psychosis. Each of these modes of internal visualization is characterized by a different intensity and duration of imaginary detail; the more intense and durable the phantom detail, the less it looks like imagination and the more it begins to look like psychosis. Mediating transitions between external alertness and internal visualization is a baseline for perceptual stability; confusing the two would be problematic. The function of internal visualization is activated by the medial temporal lobe and modulated by neurotransmitter acetylcholine; psychedelics presumably activate this function spontaneously by interrupting aminergic alertness of the forebrain.[25] If psychedelic hallucinations capitalize on the brain's capacity to produce vivid dreamlike images, we would expect the detail of a psychedelic frame to match the information profile of a dream frame; low information resolution, fleeting and erratic state data, low formal durability from frame to frame. This means that contextual information such as identity, location, and purpose would also morph and transition many times over the period of a few seconds.

If the quality of a hallucinogenic frame matches the formal quality of a dream frame, one could expect psychedelic visions to be of lower resolution than normal vision; but subjective reports indicate that multiple layers of dreaming and waking consciousness can overlap in a single frame, creating a complex overlay of both real and imagined perceptions. Being unable to separate imagination from reality is the clinical definition of psychosis, but also implies an increase in potential frame information density, which implies expanded consciousness.

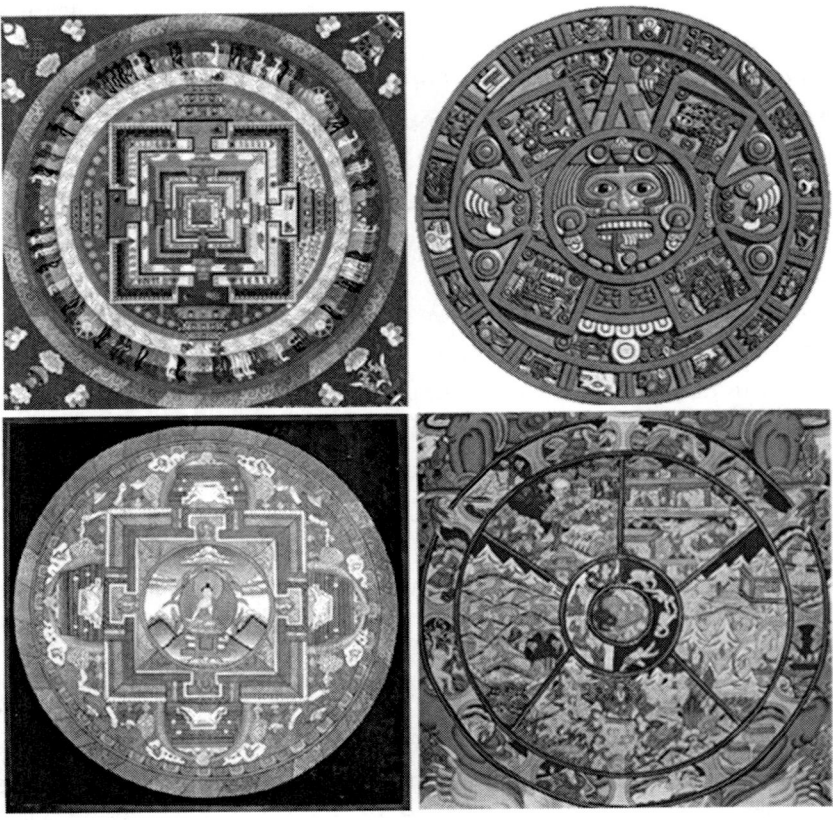

Figure 7. Mandalas and calendars representing universal harmony and knowledge. Top row: a Kalachakra time-wheel mandala; a Mesoamerican calendar. Bottom row: a mandala of the enlightened Buddha; a mandala of the Wheel of Life (Bhavacakra, or samsara). Nonlinear art embeds holographic information – such as an entire cosmology – into a single image.

The Limits of Expanded Consciousness

If the human imagination is infinite, and if psychedelics can expand the capacity of human imagination, then psychedelics can paradoxically make the infinite even more infinite. This makes sense if you accept that infinity is a linear concept which starts at zero and goes in one direction forever; but if infinity is bent into a series of repeating loops and spirals then it begins to look more like a fractal than a line, and thus more psychedelic. Human perception is linear, but humans live in a nonlinear system. One of the basic limitations of human consciousness in the inability to think exponentially; even with mathematics to assist us, envisioning and predicting exponentially complex systems is a vast conceptual hurdle. Psychedelics destabilize linear perceptions of space and time to produce fractal states of frame layering, bifurcation, and infinite frame recursion. This allows perception to become exponential, to exist in multiple states at once, much like a quantum computer that processes multiple simultaneous probabilities. If normal human imagination is bound within the limits of linear infinity, psychedelic perception is expanded to the limits of exponential or fractal infinity. Psychedelic perception presents a progressive nonlinear bifurcation of recursive self-similar information corresponding to both internal and external perceptual space. The psychedelic layering, bifurcating, and regression of internal and external perceptions creates a timeless, transpersonal perspective of a fractal rendering of time and space.[26]

The perception of seeing all time and space unfolding as a single unified function is a theme that has been reproduced in Eastern mandalas and Mesoamerican calendars for thousands of years, where a central figure sits in the center of concentric interlocking rings of reality (Fig. 7). In Sanskrit this great wheel of time is called Kalachakra (time wheel), and Kalachakra yoga emphasizes the interlocking self-similarity of body cycles and celestial cycles.[27] The description of Kalachakra overlaps with Mesoamerican cyclical calendars and spiritual themes, expressed by Maria Sabina, the Oaxacan healer who first shared the magic mushroom known as *Teonanacatl* with R. Gordon Wasson. Sabina said, "The more you go inside the world of *Teonanacatl*... you see our past and our future, which are there together as a thing already achieved, already happened... I knew and saw God: an immense clock that ticks, the spheres that go slowly around, and inside the stars, the earth, the entire universe, the day, the night... He who knows to the end the secret of *Teonanacatl* can even see that infinite clockwork."[28] This is undoubtedly a reference to Kalachakra, the great wheel of time.

Witnessing the timeless infinity of Kalachakra can be compared to Western models of Gnosticism and Hermeticism ("As Above, So Below") where the pinnacle of mystical achievement is channeling the infinite wisdom of the universal spirit;[29] or early Deist notions of a God as a great Clockmaker who set the universe in motion and let it run without intervention.[30] According to Maria Sabina's report, the subjective experience of the infinite clockwork is an end secret of psychedelic vision; this is where you arrive if you follow the process of fractal information regression to the beginning and end of all time. The thought of experiencing Kalachakra as expressed by Maria Sabina stretches the boundaries of believability, but the subjective reports of a timeless, infinite psychedelic space where the size of the universe is revealed and everything in the past and the future has already occurred is common enough to conclude that this experience is not only possible, but that it might be the end-point of expanded human consciousness. [31]

Notes and References

1. WikiPedia.org, "Visible spectrum". Internet Reference, 2010.

2. Miller RE II, Col (RET), "The Eye and Night Vision". USAF Special Report, "Night Vision Manual for the Flight Surgeon", 1992.

3. Accounts of colors seen in tryptamine hallucinations from subjective reports.

4. Hill RM, Fischer R, "Interpretation of visual space under drug-induced ergotropic and trophotropic arousal". Agents Actions, 1971 Nov;2(3):122-30.

5. Fischer R, et al., "Psilocybin-induced contraction of nearby visual space". Agents Actions, 1970 Aug;1(4):190-7.

6. Fischer R, "Effects of psychodysleptic drug psilocybin on visual perception. Changes in brightness preference". Experientia, 1969 Feb 15;25(2):166-9.

7. Accounts of seeing auras taken from subjective reports. Casual tests to confirm spectral claims have been inconclusive.

8. Michael F. Deering, "Limits of Human Vision". Sun Microsystems, 1998.

9. WikiPedia.org, "Electroencephalography". Internet Reference, 2010.

10. WikiPedia.org, "Subliminal stimuli". Internet Reference, 2010.

11. VanRullen R, et al., "The Continuous Wagon Wheel Illusion and the 'When' Pathway of the Right Parietal Lobe: A Repetitive Transcranial Magnetic Stimulation Study". PLoS ONE 3(8): August 6, 2008.

12. WikiPedia.org, "Wagon wheel effect". Internet Reference, 2010.

13. Bach M, "Wagon-wheel effect". From Michael's Optical Illusions & Visual Phenomena. Internet Reference, 2010.

14. VanRullen, Rufin, "The continuous Wagon Wheel Illusion is object-based". Vision Research Volume 46, Issue 24, November 2006, Pages 4091-4095.

15. WikiPedia.org, "Working memory". Internet Reference, 2010.

16. See Chapter 12, "Erratic Hallucination".

17. WikiPedia.org, "Retina". Internet Reference, 2010.

18. Gutkin, Pinto, Ermentrout, "Mathematical Neuroscience: From Neurons to Circuits to Systems". Journal of Physiology - Paris 97 (2003) 209–219.

19. LeDoux, Joseph, "Synaptic Self". Viking Penguin, NY, 2002.

20. WikiPedia.org, "Peripheral drift illusion". Internet Reference, 2008.

21. WikiPedia.org, "Grid illusion". Internet Reference, 2010.

22. Pinna, Baingio, "Pinna Illusion". Scholarpedia, 4(2):6656, 2009.

23. The low rendering of human visual imagination is taken from a survey of subjective reports. The quality of internal visualization is enhanced by closing the eyes and falling into a state like meditating or daydreaming.

24. Hobson, J. Allan, "The Dream Drugstore: Chemically Altered States of Consciousness". MIT Press, 2001.

25. Hobson JA, et al., "The neuropsychology of REM sleep dreaming". NeuroReport 9:3, pR1-R14, 16 February 1998.

26. A fractal is a nonlinear algorithms that repeats a basic set of instructions to generate complex, self-similar, recurrent patterns from microscopic to macroscopic to cosmic scales.

27. WikiPedia.org, "Kalachakra". Internet Reference, 2010.

28. Schultes RE, Hofmann A, "Plants of the Gods". Healing Arts Press, Vermont, 1992.

29. WikiPedia.org, "Hermeticism". Internet Reference, 2010.

30. WikiPedia.org, "Watchmaker analogy". Internet Reference, 2010.

31. Exploring the mystical implications of Kalachakra, the great fractal time wheel, has filled many volumes and fueled many prophecies. There is a solid case to be made that Kalachakra is the pinnacle of all mystical achievement; the end of psychedelic exploration; and the endpoint of human consciousness. Since the psychedelic Godhead is a transcendent state of timeless, infinite, omniscient consciousness, it is doubtful that anything more complex or expansive can ever be experienced by the human mind, marking the functional end-point of expanded consciousness.

Figure 8. Stabilized and Destabilized Perception.

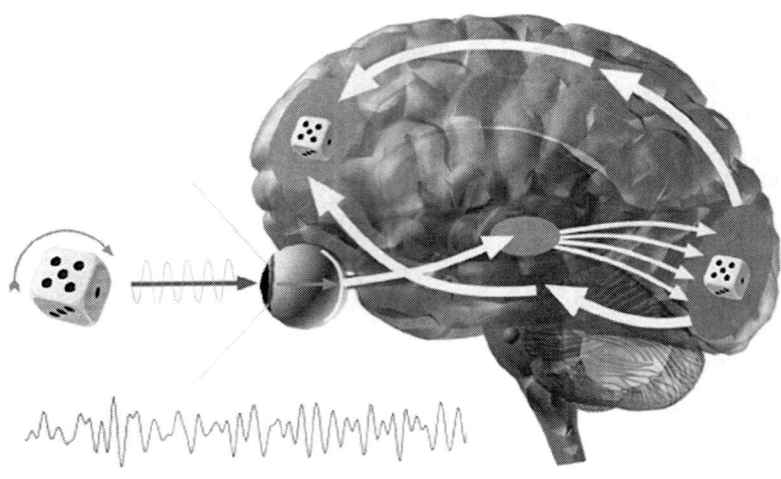

Stable perception refreshes at 15 frames per second, allowing seamless update of consciousness in the beta range of 12-30 Hz, indicated by the wave. At this refresh rate objects and textures can be rendered with high precision.

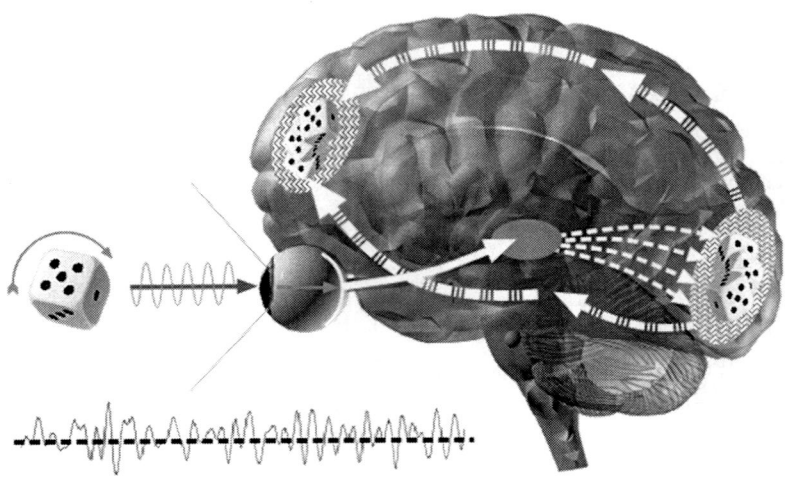

When the precise frame refresh rate of perception is interrupted, consciousness destabilizes and begins to track overlapping information from multiple receding frames. Destabilization, feedback, and latency of frame refresh creates sensory echo and complex frame interference patterns.

Chapter 06

The Control Interrupt Model of Psychedelic Action

The brain is an information processing organ that uses top-down signal modulation to control the flow of bottom-up sensory input. Feedback modulation of incoming signal is an example of self-stabilizing control in an information processing system. Using the tenets of cognition and control theory it is possible to describe a model in which hallucinogens periodically interrupt the top-down modulatory control of perception to create sensory interference patterns, multisensory frame destabilization, and altered states of consciousness.

Bottom-up Perception, Top-Down Control

What we perceive as waking consciousness is a synthesis of bottom-up sensation modified by top-down expectation and analysis.[1] Incoming sensation is gated by the top-down focus of subjective attention. Inhibitory feedback subtracts background noise while excitatory feedback resolves and amplifies salient data. This configuration describes a signal filter-amplifier with an inhibitory-excitatory feedback loop to control signal focus and content discrimination. The top-down filtering and focusing of sensory signal is an autonomic reflex and is perceptually seamless; the brain blocks background noise, transitions focus, and recognizes objects without disrupting subjective frame continuity. Without the ability to control incoming sensory signal with feedback, perception would become under-constrained, distracted, overloaded, exuberant, and error-prone. Under-constrained internal sensory noise entering into multisensory awareness would be perceived as hallucination.

Constraint, Control, and Feedback Inhibition

Feedback excitation is applied in sensory circuits to amplify salient input, but the majority of the brain's feedback circuits are inhibitory, meaning that human consciousness is more constrained than unconstrained. In dynamical information processing systems, signal constraint and error correction is applied through negative feedback to subtract or cancel perturbation and noise entering the signal circuit; this is known as control theory. In sensory networks, such as the layers of the cortex or the retina, fast inhibition is applied laterally to boost contrast discrimination in line detail; this is called lateral inhibition. Fast inhibition in the cortex can also be applied from the bottom-up as well as laterally, this is called the synaptic triad of fast inhibition. Inhibition can also be applied from the top-down, allowing the logical cortex to filter or ignore noisy input from the thalamus; this is called top-down feedback inhibition, and it is typically tonic, meaning top-down feedback is inhibitory over many consecutive spike trains to control extended periods of channeled focus. When the brain is alert and focused, this means it is highly constrained by inhibitory feedback.

When people express their fears about psychedelics, the most commonly voiced concern is the fear of losing control. Common entheogenic wisdom states that you must relinquish control and submit to the experience to get the most out of psychedelics. Holding onto control causes negative experiences and amplifies anxiety. Metaphors for control and submission are applied to psychedelics because hallucinogens subvert various forms of feedback control, allowing perception and behavior to become unconstrained and unpredictable. Extreme states of under-constrained perception would include sensory saturation, sensory echo, synesthesia, hallucination, disorientation, and confusion. Extreme states of under-constrained behavior would include mania, hysteria, paranoia, euphoria, and as the system becomes totally overloaded, catatonia.

Loss of feedback restraint in a dynamical information processing system causes output to become exuberant and unpredictable; this is called deterministic chaos, or chaos in deterministic systems. In order for a perceptual system to transition from a linear to a chaotic or nonlinear state, negative feedback control must be removed or subverted by a periodic driving force. If control is entirely removed then perception becomes totally unconstrained, leaving a system that is quickly overloaded with too much information. If control is placed in a partially removed state, or in a toggled superposition where it is alternately in control and not in control over the period of a rapid oscillation, then the constraints of linear sensory throughput will bifurcate into a nonlinear spectrum of multi-stable output with signal complexity correlating to the method of control interruption.

The Control Interrupt Model of Psychedelic Action

Before the mind can start hallucinating, the top-down modulatory control of consciousness must first be interrupted. Interrupting top-down control of consciousness allows the mind to destabilize into novel information processing configurations. When top-down control of waking consciousness is destabilized, neural oscillators in the brain will spontaneously organize into coherence with the most energetic local drivers. This process can be described in terms of oscillator entrainment and resonance; when the modulatory driver maintaining global oscillator coherence is interrupted, uncoupled oscillators will naturally fall into synchrony with most energetic periodic drivers in the environment.[2] In this state, the normally inflexible configurations of consciousness and perception become extensible and open to the influence of environmental feedback. This explains why psychedelics create synesthesia or cross-sensory representations of energetic sensory drivers, and why set and setting have a profound influence on the tone and content of a psychedelic experience.

When top-down modulatory control of consciousness is interrupted, the seamless nature of multisensory perception degrades and the subject begins to experience hallucinations (Fig. 8). Early indicators of modulatory interruption include periodic high-frequency distortion or noise in sensory networks. In tactile networks this periodic interruption may be felt as parasthesia, or phantom tingling and pulsating; in visual networks it may be perceived as phosphenes, or strobing or flickering of light intensity, possibly fast enough to produce geometric hallucinations; in audio networks it may be perceived as tinnitus, ringing, humming, buzzing, or tones that cycle up and down in pitch. These are all descriptions of field-based hallucinations generated in response to periodic interruptions along multisensory signal pathways. The speed and intensity of the control interrupt, and thus the speed and intensity of the hallucinations, are a direct result of the hallucinogen's pharmacodynamics and method of ingestion.

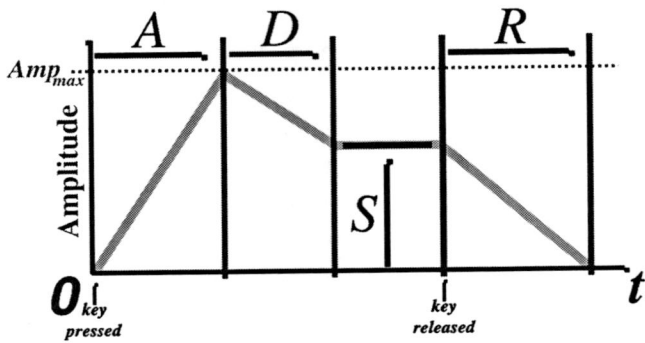

Figure 9. Using an Attack-Decay-Sustain-Release (ADSR) envelope we can model the intensity of hallucinogenic interrupt for any drug. From WikiPedia.

Control Interrupt Envelopes

Using control interruption as the source of hallucinogenesis, we can model hallucinogenic frame distortion of multisensory perception the same way we model sound waves produced by synthesizers; by plotting the attack, decay, sustain, and release (ADSR envelope) of the interruption as it effects consciousness (Fig. 9).[3,4] For example, nitrous oxide (N_2O) inhalation alters consciousness in such a way that all perceptual frames arise and fall with a predictable "wah-wah-wah" time signature. The throbbing "wah-wha-wah" of the N_2O experience is a stable standing wave formation that begins when the molecule hits the neural network and ends when it is metabolized, but for the duration of N_2O action the "wah-wah-wah" completely penetrates all modes of sensory awareness with a strobe-like intensity. The N_2O sensation is often described as a soft tingling, throbbing, or buzzing that grows to consume all sensation.

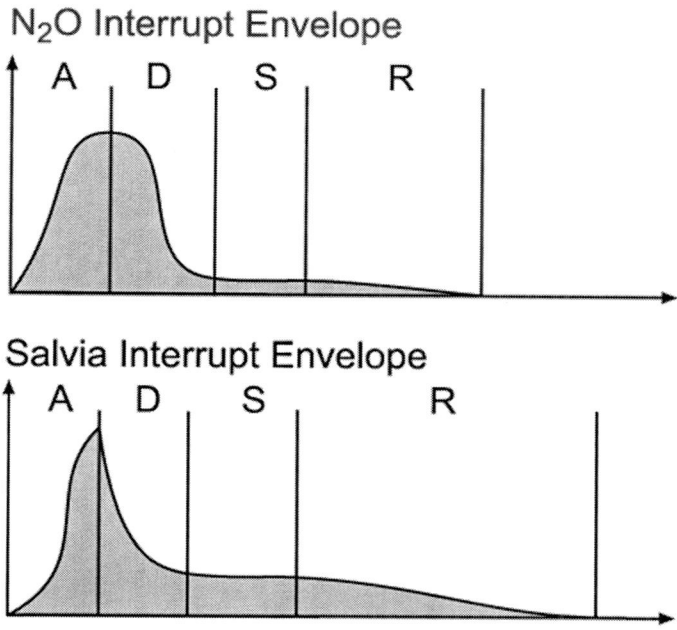

Figure 10. Modeling the interrupt envelope for N_2O and Salvia we can see N_2O has a hard but rounded attack and decay. In contrast Salvia has a slightly faster and more intense ADSR profile, describing a slightly more biting and disorienting effect on multisensory perception.

Taking into account the subjective reports of N_2O action, the periodic interrupt of N_2O's "wah-wah-wah" can be modeled as a perceptual wave ambiguity that toggles back and forth between saturated consciousness and semi-consciousness at roughly 8 to 11 frames-per-second, or @8-11 Hz (hertz).[5] Consciousness rises at the peak of each "wah" and diminishes in the valleys in between, growing in sustained intensity with each cycle until the subject passes out. On sub-anesthetic doses, N_2O creates a looping effect where frame content overlaps into the following frame, causing a perceptual cascade similar to fractal regression. We can thus model the interrupt envelope of N_2O as having a rounded attack, fast decay, low sustain, medium release, with an interrupt frequency of @8-11 Hz. Any psychoactive substance with a similar frequency and shape of interrupt envelope will produce results that feel similar to the N_2O experience (Fig. 10). For instance,

Smoked *Salvia divinorum* (vaporized Salvinorin A&B, or Salvia) has an interrupt envelope similar to N_2O, except Salvia has a slightly faster interrupt frequency (@12-15 Hz), a harder attack, a slightly longer decay, a more intense sustain, and a slightly longer release.[6] These slight changes in the frequency and shape of interrupt envelope cause Salvia to feel more physically intense, more hallucinatory, and more disorienting than N_2O, even though they share a similar throbbing or tingling sensation along the same pathways and frequency range.

Using interrupt envelopes we can contrast smoked Salvia or inhaled N_2O with vaporized DMT (N,N-dimethyltryptamine), which when smoked has similar onset and duration to both substances but very different hallucinogenic effects. Unlike the slow throbbing periodicity of N_2O or Salvia, vaporized DMT produces an interrupt frequency associated with a high-pitched carrier wave and high-speed frame flicker (24-30+ Hz). The frequency of DMT's interrupt is so rapid the entire body ramps up in panicked response to the new driver. The rate of DMT's visual frame flicker is fast enough to instantly produce geometric hallucinations and fully realized animations.[7] Taking these subjective effects into account we can model DMT's interrupt envelope as having a moderate attack, long decay, medium sustain, long release, and high frequency (24-30+ Hz). The moderate attack means DMT's perceptual frame interference is less of a physical throbbing than N_2O, but because of a higher frequency and longer frame release the rendering of DMT hallucination is more fluid, detailed, seamlessly aliased, and fades longer over a higher number of frames.

The interrupt envelopes modeled here are approximate and based on reported subjective effects, but may also give some insight into the pharmacodynamics of each substance.[8] Following the logic of the Control Interrupt Model, it can be assumed that each hallucinogen has a unique interrupt envelope based on receptor affinity, receptor density, rate of metabolism, and so on, and each unique interrupt envelope creates a distinct type of interference pattern in multisensory perception. The interrupt envelope for any substance will also change if the substance is ingested orally as opposed to vaporized or injected; the speed of absorption into the bloodstream will naturally affect the intensity of ADSR values. This is why each psychedelic can produce unique sensations and hallucinations, and why each psychedelic can produce subtle variations in the speed and intensity of hallucination depending on method of ingestion.[9]

By modeling the interrupt envelope of a psychoactive substance it is possible to accurately predict its subjective results on multisensory perception. Non-drug sources of hallucination, such as those caused by psychosis, deprivation, fever, or schizophrenia, may also have unique and quantifiable control interrupt envelopes related to erratic multisensory frame modulation.

Control Interrupt and Shamanism

If consciousness must have a top-down control frequency to remain stable, and psychedelics produce a periodic interruption of this control frequency, then the interaction between the perceptual control frequency and the periodic interruption can be described as a wave interference pattern in global oscillator coherence. Subjects on moderate doses of psychedelics can override the hallucinogenic interrupt and retain global coherence via energetic physical movement or repetitive behaviors like chanting or dancing. Conversely, if the subject lies motionless, then the interruption fully destabilizes alert consciousness into a depersonalized dreamlike trance.[10] These reports indicate that even though psychedelics destabilize top-down modulatory control of consciousness, feedback control and linear system stability can be entrained back into coherence via external periodic drivers, including rhythmic motor activity, drumming, singing, chanting, rocking back and forth, dancing, and so on. It is no accident that these are also the basic formal elements of shamanic ritual.

In physical terms, the shaman is the primary energetic driver, or resonator, stabilizing attractors within the chaotic hallucinogenic interference pattern created in the consciousness of the subject. In the mathematics of nonlinear dynamics, this phase-locking action is similar to deterministic chaos seen when entraining limit cycles in a forced Van der Pol oscillator.[11] By prescribing a psychedelic substance, the shaman introduces the control frequency interrupt, and through ritual craft and showmanship the shaman applies harmonic interference to navigate and influence the tone and texture of the trip. By mixing the hallucinogenic control interrupt with a harmonic periodic driver the shaman can entrain expanded states of consciousness and manipulate the subject's mind with high precision. The precision wave-based manipulation of neural oscillators within the psychedelic state can be called applied psychedelic science, physical shamanism, or Shamanism in the Age of Reason.

Notes and References

1. Corlett PR, Frith CD, Fletcher PC, "From drugs to deprivation: a Bayesian framework for understanding models of psychosis". Psychopharmacology (Berl). 2009 November; 206(4): 515–530.

2. WikiPedia.org, "Entrainment (Physics)". Internet Reference, 2009.

3. ADSR envelopes were chosen as the best available shorthand for approximating differences in the tone and texture of each hallucinogen as it interrupts consciousness. Arguably a more precise model could be employed, but using ADSR compresses a longer discussion on how to precisely model intensity and onset of subjective hallucinogenic effects.

4. WikiPedia.org, "ADSR envelope". Internet Reference, 2009.

5. N_2O interrupt envelope is an approximation based on subjective reports.

6. Salvia interrupt envelope is an approximation based on subjective reports.

7. DMT interrupt envelope is an approximation based on subjective reports.

8. Most receptor interactions occur on the order of microseconds, so attempting to model pharmacodynamics based on rate of subjective frame interruption may be impossible, or require complex statistical interpretations.

9. ADSR envelopes will change slightly for any substance depending on dose and speed of absorption into the bloodstream, but beyond that they may also change depending on the purity of hallucinogen. For instance, if an LSD experience is described as "clean", this means the hallucinogenic interrupt is so subtle that it is almost invisible; this also implies purity of the LSD. In contrast, when an LSD experience is described as "dirty" or "jagged", this means the interrupt induces transitions in consciousness that are abrupt and unpleasant; this also implies the LSD is adulterated or has not been sufficiently purified. It is widely accepted that if one batch of LSD induces a soft interrupt envelope with a wiggly and sensual attack, that same LSD should produce similar result for everyone. The same would be true for LSD that produces a jagged and abrupt attack. If a pure sample set could be acquired and tested, it may be possible to model precise interrupt frequencies and ADSR envelopes for every known psychoactive substance.

10. Reports taken from subjective accounts and corroborated over multiple subjects and experiences.

11. Kanamaru, T., "Van der Pol oscillator", *Scholarpedia*, 2(1), 2202, (2007).

Chapter 07

Psychedelic Pharmacology

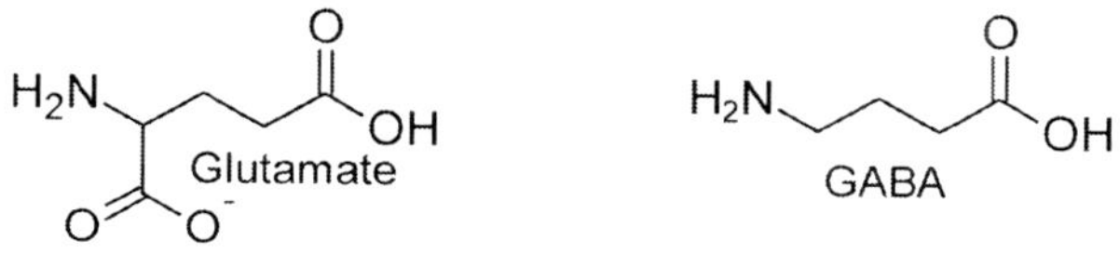

Figure 11. Glutamate ad GABA, the neural messengers for go and stop. Glutamate excites neurons and promotes spiking, GABA inhibits spike trains.

Sensory signal traveling through the brain is mediated by glutamate, an excitatory chemical messenger. Sensory signal is filtered by GABA, an inhibitory messenger GABA (Fig. 11). The precise spike timing of these messengers is tuned by neuromodulators, which synchronize spiking across the entire brain. Most hallucinogens are structurally similar to the modulators which tune global spike timing, such as serotonin (5-HT), norepinephrine (noradrenaline), and dopamine (DA) (Fig. 12). All of these chemicals are classified as amines, meaning that they have a nitrogen (N^+) containing amino group hanging off a root carbon ring. This nitrogen structure is the key element in any amino acid, carrying the energy needed for metabolic processes which do work. Since these transmitter chemicals have only one nitrogen group they are called monoamines, and they are the essential messengers of the aminergic neuromodulatory system.

Monoamines entering the bloodstream are normally kept out of the brain by the blood-brain-barrier, but psychedelic molecules have a neutral charge so they are able to pass. When these amine crystals pass through the blood-brain barrier they brush against neural receptor sites; if the receptors are a good fit then the crystals get stuck for a short period of time. The bonding of amine ligands to serotonin and dopamine receptors is where psychedelic action begins.[1,2]

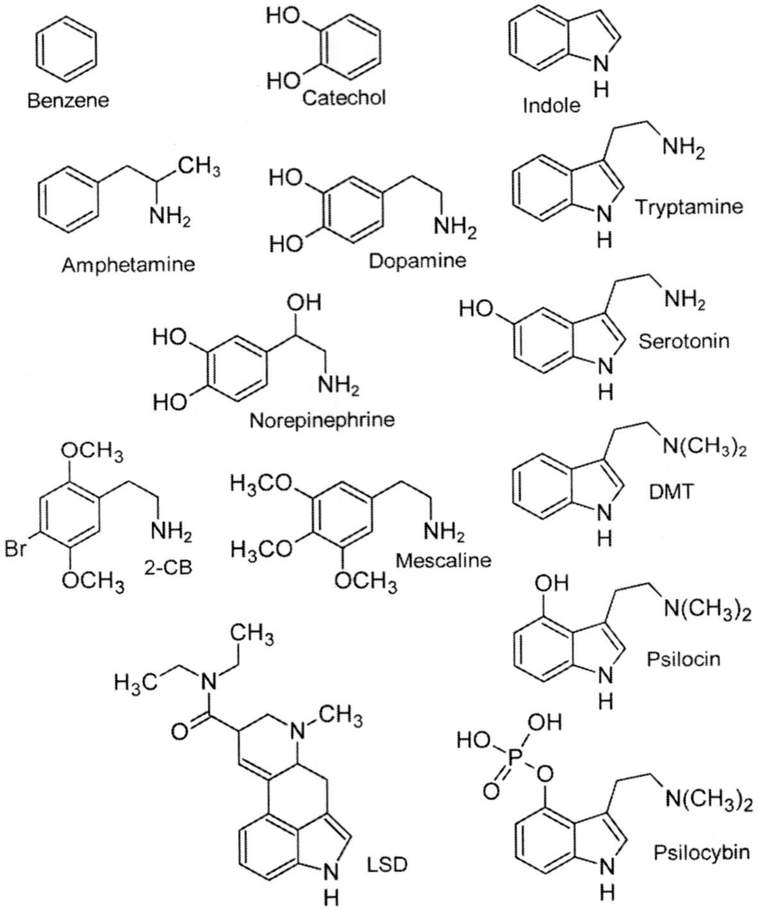

Figure 12: Psychedelic amines look very much like the endogenous neurotransmitters serotonin, norepinephrine, and dopamine. On the left are the adrenal-promoting catecholamines, amphetamines, and phenethylamines; on the right are the indoleamines, also called tryptamines, and their hallucinogenic counterparts. LSD, a synthesized molecule, is also an indoleamine, but is more structurally engineered than its organic counterparts.

Serotonin and the Tryptamines

Because of depressive mood disorders and pharmaceuticals like Prozac, the most well known neuromodulator is serotonin, or 5-HT (5-hydroxytryptamine). 5-HT is essential to many basic brain functions, linked to mood, depression, contentment, learning, anxiety, sleep, appetite, and the regulation of involuntary smooth muscles that control blood pressure and digestion. Serotonin is an indoleamine and a variant of tryptamine, which is the most basic of all the indoleamines and the structural starting point for DMT (N,N-dimethyltryptamine), 5-MeO-DMT, psilocin, psilocybin, DPT, AMT, and most psychedelic drugs with acronyms ending in T (which stands for Tryptamine). LSD is also an indoleamine, but it is larger and more complex than organic indoleamines, and is in many ways structurally unique.

Dopamine and the Phenethylamines

Working in concert with serotonin is the neuromodulator dopamine (3-hydroxytyramine). Dopamine is synthesized from L-DOPA and is instrumental in modulating salient attention, motivational response, and fine motor control. Dopamine is central to the reward system, and dopamine release is stimulated by recreational drugs, food, gambling, sex, and physical risk taking. Dopamine imbalances are linked Parkinson's disease, ADD, compulsive risk behavior, and psychosis. The role of dopamine interruption is relevant to psychedelic activity in many aspects; psychedelics may affect sensuality and motor control, and may facilitate psychosis, mania, and compulsive behaviors.

Amphetamines and the phenethylamine group of psychedelics (mescaline, 2-CB, MDA, MDMA, and so on) are more structurally similar to dopamine, epinephrine, and norepinephrine, which are also monoamines but sometimes referred to as catecholamines since they are based on the single catechol ring structure. Epinephrine and norepinephrine are referred to as stress hormones because they prime the body's adrenal production and energy response to stress and danger. The phenethylamines and catecholamines all have the six-carbon benzene ring backbone, simpler than the dual-ring tryptamine structure, with at least one amine group. The simplest form of this molecule is called phenethylamine, and is similar to amphetamine.

In very general terms, the phenethylamine psychedelics are said to be more energetic, sensual, empathogenic, or entactogenic, while tryptamine psychedelics are thought to be more hallucinogenic, disorienting, and somatically heavy. These descriptions are very broad, but this is the popular distinction made between the two major classes of psychedelics.

Neuromodulators and Global Brain States

Serotonin, dopamine, and the other monoamines don't cause neurons to fire, they instead tune the spiking rate of neurons, which means they adjust global network polarity over time to make neural assemblies more or less responsive to stimulus. Serotonin and dopamine are projected into higher areas of the brain from nuclei in the brainstem and middle brain, meaning they are primal signaling mechanisms for modulating many areas of the brain simultaneously. The axons from these aminergic clusters reach upward to many areas of the cortex, affecting the thalamus (sensory filter), amygdala (fear and survival), hypothalamus (homeostatic regulator), hippocampus (memory and learning), and neocortex (sensory and logic processing). Neuromodulators synchronize the neural response to incoming stimulus and keep local competing brain circuits functioning smoothly and in unison. These neuromodulators produce a one-way bottom-up effect, which means they are switched on and off reflexively and unconsciously by glands in the brainstem and basal forebrain in direct response to internal conditions or external stimulus. With neuromodulators the brainstem can exert global homeostatic control over organism mood and behavior. The effect of the aminergic modulators projected upward by the brainstem are tonic, which means their signaling effects are sticky and persist over the duration of many incoming spike trains.

Generally serotonin is thought to have a polarizing effect on neurons, making them less likely to fire and thus having an overall relaxing effect on the brain. This is why many depression and anxiety remedies focus on increasing the supply of serotonin; to decrease anxiety and increase satisfaction. If we assume psychedelics are mimics for neurotransmitters and apply this analogy to DMT, we would expect DMT to have a calming effect on the brain because it looks similar to serotonin. But a flood of DMT does not calm the brain, it makes it hallucinate. Since DMT binds to the same receptor sites as serotonin but does not produce a relaxing effect, it would be logical to assume that DMT is a 5-HT antagonist, meaning it blocks serotonin and depolarizes neurons, making them more excitable. This is not the case. There are many different types of 5-HT receptors, some inhibit neural activity and some promote neural activity. Like most hallucinogens, DMT is classified as a selective $5\text{-}HT_{2A}$ partial or full agonist; also active at other 5-HT subtypes, at DA receptors, at adrenal receptors, at Sigma-1 receptors, and at tertiary amine receptors. This means that DMT is active at many receptor sites and can mimic the agonistic functions of serotonin with varying affinity and efficacy.

$5\text{-}HT_{2A}$ partial agonism can be described as a subtle form of aminergic modulatory signal interference. In the most general case it can be assumed that psychedelic activity is due to interference at 5-HT receptor subtypes. In more specific cases we can assume that visual hallucinogenic effect is associated with $5\text{-}HT_{2A}$ and $5\text{-}HT_{2C}$ receptor interaction. Somatic heaviness and dreaminess is associated with broader aminergic interaction; and more sensual, entactogenic, or compulsive effects are associated with dopamine and adrenergic receptor interaction. Psychedelics can have a wide affinity and interact as partial or full agonists at multiple receptor subtypes to produce a wide range of effects.

Because psychedelics are full or partial agonists acting on the same modulatory pathways as 5-HT, the synergistic interaction between these competing agonists can be described in terms of a modulatory wave interference pattern. Agonistic interference at 5-HT subtypes promotes disinhibition and cross-excitability between feedback-coupled assemblies in the brain. Excitation and loss of feedback inhibition in the circuits responsible for processing sensation and perception lead to spontaneous self-sustaining feedback hallucinations. Prolonged states of feedback excitation between the circuits which process perception and memory leads to infinite working memory regression and expanded states of psychedelic consciousness.

Molecular Shape, Receptor Affinity, MAO Metabolism

The strength and duration of the bond a ligand forms with a receptor is referred to as receptor affinity or potency, and is described in terms of pharmacodynamics. The higher the affinity, the stronger and longer the ligand bonds with a receptor, thus influencing neural activity. Research has shown that 5-HT$_{2A}$ receptor affinity is an accurate measure of the potency of any psychedelic compound; the higher the affinity the higher the potency and psychedelic effect.[4,5] Another thing we know is that the conformational shape of the amine determines how long the molecule takes to metabolize and how sticky it will be at 5-HT receptor types.[6] For instance, the amine tail of LSD is different from other tryptamines; it is long, complex, and connects back to the benzene ring, keeping it rigid instead of flexible like most amino groups or substitutions. Designer amines with a similarly rigid molecular structure have also shown a marked increase in psychedelic potency.[7]

Using this information it can be assumed that the unique structure of LSD is what makes it so potent; giving it a high affinity across a wider range of receptor types; making it more difficult to metabolize; and giving it a broader range of effect over a longer duration. DMT also binds to a wide variety of 5-HT receptor types, but it is smaller and metabolizes very quickly. When DMT is taken with a monoamine-oxidase inhibitor (MAOi) in an ayahuasca mixture, the enzymes which metabolize DMT are blocked, making the hallucinogenic effects of DMT orally active and longer lasting. Adding an MAOi to any tryptamine psychedelic will make it nearly twice as hallucinogenic.[8] These few pieces of pharmacology tell us that the efficacy of modulatory interruption, or psychedelic potency, can be somewhat predicted by molecular shape, the rigidity of the molecular structure, and speed of metabolic pathways. If metabolic pathways are degraded by synergistic dosing, as in an ayahuasca mixture, then the potency of the drug increases over the duration of effect in direct proportion to the latency of metabolism.

5HT-	1A	1B	1D	1E	2A	2B	2C	5A	6	7	D1	a2A	a2B	a2C
2C-E	2.91	3.00	3.54	2.60	3.76	4.00	3.38	0.00	1.93	2.77	0.00	2.71	2.91	3.44
2C-B	2.75	3.11	3.71	3.05	3.69	4.00	3.18	0.00	2.63	2.81	0.00	2.64	2.31	3.12
LSD	3.73	4.00	3.70	2.62	3.54	3.11	3.11	3.64	3.75	3.77	2.34	2.93	0.00	0.00
DOI	0.00	2.31	3.00	2.66	3.44	3.13	4.00	0.00	2.34	1.90	1.67	3.79	3.13	2.88
DMT	0.00	0.00	3.91	3.28	2.58	0.00	3.42	3.16	3.35	4.00	3.51	2.75	3.53	3.53
Psilocin	2.88	2.19	3.40	3.03	2.14	4.00	2.52	2.83	2.82	2.82	3.37	1.36	1.57	1.03
5MDMT	4.00	2.41	3.48	1.72	0.98	0.69	1.55	1.84	2.73	3.69	2.38	0.00	0.86	1.57
DiPT	4.00	0.00	2.51	0.00	0.00	3.48	0.00	0.00	0.00	0.00	0.00	0.00	2.62	2.68
Mescaline	3.61	0.00	0.00	3.16	0.00	3.97	0.00	0.00	0.00	0.00	0.00	2.92	0.00	4.00
MDMA	0.00	0.00	0.00	0.00	0.00	3.64	0.00	0.00	0.00	0.00	0.00	2.94	3.09	3.21
6-F-DMT	2.81	3.07	3.66	2.74	2.47	3.93	2.58	2.43	4.00	3.80	2.67	0.00	2.99	3.24
Lisuride	4.00	2.27	0.00	0.00	2.74	3.01	0.00	2.99	2.61	2.64	0.00	3.22	3.78	3.88
4C-T-2	2.04	0.00	0.00	1.77	3.33	4.00	3.09	2.56	0.00	2.18	0.00	0.00	0.00	0.00

Table 1: Popular psychedelic drug affinities across aminergic receptor targets listed in order of 5-HT$_{2A}$ receptor affinity, with dopamine (D1) and adrenal receptors on the right. A value of 4.00 indicates high affinity at that target; any value under 2.00 should be considered imperceptible. Three non-psychedelic control molecules are listed at the bottom for comparison. From Ray, 2010.[3]

Breadth of Psychedelic Receptor Binding

Table 1 lists the binding strength of popular psychedelic drugs at many 5-HT receptor sites, listed in order of 5-HT$_{2A}$ affinity.[3] This table should be an accurate representation of hallucinogenic potency of various psychedelics in descending order. From subjective reports all substances at the top of this list are very hallucinogenic, but DMT, which is often considered to be the most hallucinogenic, actually falls somewhere in the middle. If we also look at 5-HT$_{2C}$ affinity, which is implicated in hallucination, we can see that all substances at the top of the list also have high 5-HT$_{2C}$ affinity, with DMT and DOI having slightly higher affinity than the rest. 5-HT$_7$ receptor affinity, which stimulates cAMP activity and the reward system, also seems to be implicated in overall transcendent psychedelic action, with the mystically popular DMT, 5-MeO-DMT, and LSD topping the affinity list for these receptors.

In contrast, there are four non-visual psychedelics at the bottom of the list, 5-MeO-DMT, DiPT, Mescaline, and MDMA. These substances have very poor $5\text{-HT}_{2A,2C}$ affinity, but all have a high 5-HT_{2B} and adrenal affinity; this indicates they are effective at stimulating serotonin production, cardiovascular activity, and acute sensuality. 5-HT_{2B} affinity is quite high for all samples in this list with the exception of DMT and 5-MeO-DMT, making 5-HT_{2B} affinity a good indicator for purely sensual or entactogenic effect. It is interesting to note that DiPT, Mescaline, and 5-MeO-DMT all have a high 5-HT_{1A} affinity, which is generally thought to work in contrast to 5-HT_{2A} agonism to promote well-being and satisfaction. DiPT is unusual because it produces distinct audio hallucinations and little or no visual hallucinations, and predictably does not bond with $5\text{-HT}_{2A,2C}$ receptors implicated in visual hallucination. By analyzing this affinity table it seems possible to predict the relative potency and effect of any hallucinogen based solely on binding profiles, though the three control molecules at the bottom of the list (6-F-DMT, Lisuride, 4C-T-2) are reportedly non-hallucinogenic despite high 5-HT receptor promiscuity; this is likely because they are not active as agonists, they are antagonists, or their binding profiles are not synergistic and somehow cancel each other out.

Dissociatives, Anticholinergics, Other Hallucinogens

Psychedelic tryptamines and phenethylamines are not the only hallucinogens, but all hallucinogens work by interrupting sensory processing pathways. Hallucinogenic dissociatives like ketamine (special K), phencyclidine (PCP), and dextromethorphan (DXM) block NMDA glutamate sensory signaling pathways; these pathways mediate fast sensory signal projection through the brain. Anticholinergic deliriants like scopolamine and atropine interrupt cholinergic modulation of memory, recall, and dreaming; these pathways mediate the smooth input and output of memory from the hippocampus. *Salvia divinorum* interrupts kappa-Opioid tactile sensory pathways; these pathways mediate pain, gravity awareness, and sensation for determining physical orientation in space. Depressants like GHB and alcohol activate inhibitory GABA pathways, pathways which dampen and slow smooth sensory throughput. Nitrous Oxide (N_2O) is the simplest and perhaps the most promiscuous of all hallucinogens, worming its way in between a number of rudimentary signaling pathways to produce anesthetic tingling, dissociation, and out-of-body emergence. Although the pharmacological targets of hallucinogens may differ, in all cases perceptual distortion is linked directly to interruption of seamless multisensory signaling and representation across the cortex. Any drug which interrupts pathways of multisensory signaling or binding will be considered psychedelic or hallucinogenic at high enough doses, which is why so many different types of plants and chemicals can be uniquely hallucinogenic across many different receptor targets.

Notes and References

1. Snyder S, "Drugs and The Brain". Scientific American Books, 1986.

2. Cooper JR, et al., "The Biochemical Basis of Neuropharmacology". Oxford University Press, NY, 7th ed., 1996.

3. Ray TS, "Psychedelics and the Human Receptorome". PLoS One. 2010; 5(2): e9019.

4. Glennon RA, et al., "Evidence for 5-HT2 involvement in the mechanism of action of hallucinogenic agents". Life Sci. 1984 Dec 17;35(25):2505-11.

5. Sadzot B, et al., "Hallucinogenic drug interactions at human brain 5-HT2 receptors: implications for treating LSD-induced hallucinogenesis". Psychopharmacology (Berl). 1989;98(4):495-9.

6. McLean TH, Parrish JC, Braden MR, Marona-Lewicka D, Gallardo-Godoy A, Nichols DE, "1-Aminomethylbenzocycloalkanes: conformationally-restricted hallucinogenic phenethylamine analogues as functionally-selective 5-HT2A receptor agonists". J Med Chem. 2006 Sep 21;49(19):5794-803.

7. Sattelkau T, "An Interview with Dave Nichols". Trip Magazine, V5, Spring 2000, p 42.

8. Subjective reports of taking an MAO inhibitor with psychedelic tryptamines such as DMT, psilocybin, LSD, and 5-MeO-DMT confirm that the addition of an MAOi increases potency and hallucination by an order of magnitude. MAOi potentiation can come from plant sources, such as the harmala alkaloids found in *Peganum harmala* seeds and *Bandisteriopsis caapi* vine, but is particularly intense with a pharmaceutical source like moclobemide.

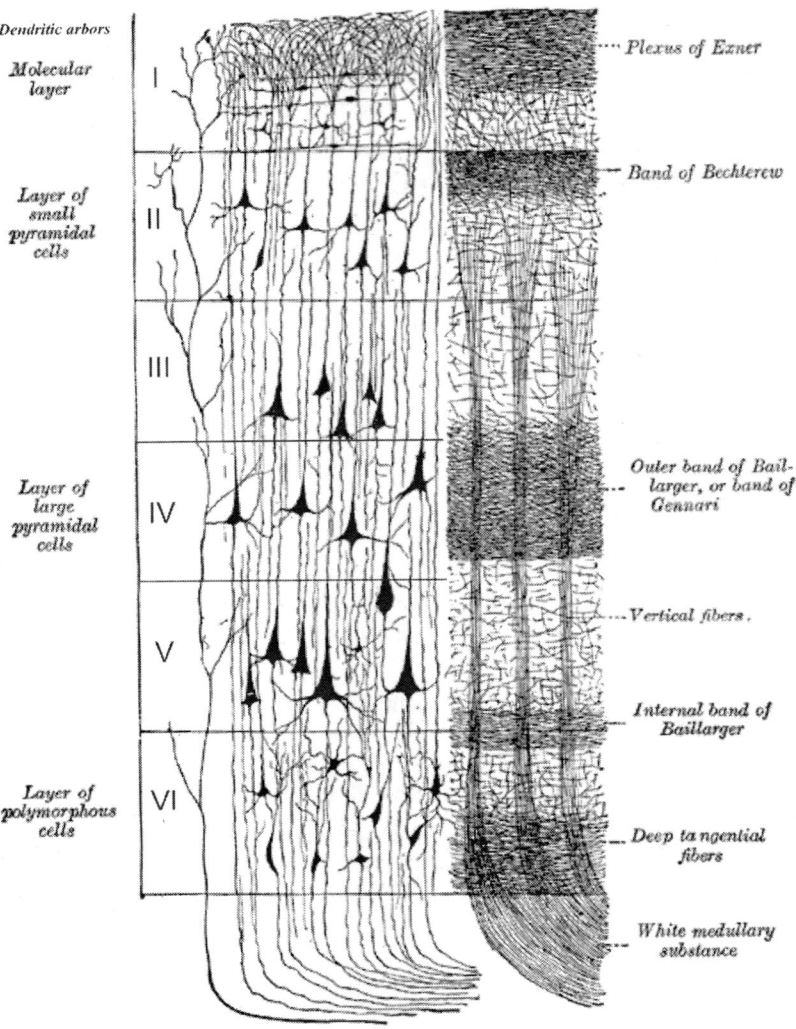

Figure 13. Layers of the neocortex. Sensory signal rises from the thalamus through intermediary cortical layers to the dendritic arbors at the top layer, the very outer membrane of the cortex, where the highest density of 5-HT$_{2A}$ receptors are expressed. The dendrite arbors in layer I connect back down to the large layer V pyramidal cells, which bind multisensory data via lateral projections, recurrent ascending projections, and reciprocal thalamocortical feedback loops. From Grey's Anatomy, modified.

Chapter 08

5-HT$_{2A}$ Agonism and Multisensory Binding

Most visual hallucinogens are active as full or partial agonists at the 5-HT$_{2A}$ receptor subtype, and all produce similar visual hallucinations that are immediately recognizable as psychedelic.[1] Although the 5-HT$_{2A}$ receptor subtype is not the only receptor implicated in hallucinogenesis,[2] it is one of the most studied hallucinogenic targets and offers some insights into the nature of psychedelic action. 5-HT$_{2A}$ receptors are ubiquitous throughout the nervous system, found in the sensory cortex, the frontal cortex, the olfactory cortex, the basal ganglia, the cerebellum, the hippocampus, thalamic nuclei, brainstem nuclei, sensory neurons, platelets, fibroblasts, intestines, smooth muscles, and cardiovascular systems.[3,4,5,6] By following the pathways of 5-HT$_{2A}$ modulated signal transduction through the human organism it is possible to extrapolate that psychedelic experience is not limited to mere hallucination, but is instead a complex multi-layered experience integrated throughout all biological signaling systems.

The layering of cellular signaling systems mediated by 5-HT provides a framework for viewing the 5-HT$_{2A}$ pathway as a primary modulator for homeostatic regulation of multisensory awareness, behavior, and learning.[7] 5-HT$_{2A}$ receptor agonists, also known as hallucinogens, promote disinhibition and excitability in 5-HT mediated pathways, indicating that psychedelic action is the product of spontaneous excitation and self-sustaining feedback in 5-HT mediated signaling pathways. The most obvious effects of 5-HT$_{2A}$ agonism are real-time perceptual distortions, or hallucination, but given the wide distribution of these receptors, there are also bound to be more subtle holistic effects on respiration, metabolism, cellular activity, memory, learning, and long term behavior.

5-HT$_{2A}$ receptor mechanics

The 5-HT$_{2A}$ receptor is a G protein-coupled receptor (GPCR), which means it does not activate ion channels or directly alter cell polarity, but instead sets off a chain reaction of intracellular signaling systems involving phosphatidylinositol (PI) hydrolysis, the production of inositol trisphosphate (IP$_3$), the release of calcium (Ca^{2+}), and the activation of protein kinase C (PKC) as well as various mitogen-activated protein kinases (MAPK).[6,8,9,25] PKC regulates a variety of cellular functions at the membrane, including signal transduction, receptor desensitization, and synaptic formation and strengthening responsible for learning and memory.[10] MAPK regulates fundamental intracellular functions in the cytoplasm and nucleus such as gene expression, proliferation, cell growth, and survival.[26] It is interesting to note that Salvinorin A, another potent hallucinogen, also stimulates PKC and MAPK signaling pathways via kappa-Opioid receptors.[28,29,30] These receptor-mediated secondary pathways undoubtedly play a role in psychedelic neuroplasticity and cellular regeneration,[27] but the stimulation of secondary messengers is not always necessary for hallucination and psychedelic effect.

Layer V pyramidal cells and perceptual binding

In the human brain the highest density of 5-HT$_{2A}$ receptors are expressed on the dendrites of cortical layer V pyramidal cells,[3,4,5,6,8] and the highest density of layer V dendrites project upward into the dendrite arbors of cortical layer I, the very outward surface of the brain (Fig. 13). 5-HT$_{2A}$ receptors in the dendritic arbors of pyramid cells are primarily responsible for modulating asynchronous (late) glutamate release in the wake of strong incoming spike trains,[1,11,12] presumably for enhanced top-down aliasing, latent reconstruction, and memory imprinting of salient sensory data.[13] Sensory signal rising to the dendrites of the cortical surface encodes a highly detailed reconstruction of external perception for latent real-time analysis and progressive perceptual filling. Multiple layers of the neocortex have descending columnar dendrites or ascending recurrent axon collaterals to provide real-time sensory feedback to latent apical rendering layers, allowing a seamless representation of perceptual motion to be synchronized across the cortex. Cortical layer V neurons receiving input through apical dendrites are one of the primary conduits for binding coherent sensory perception across the entire cortical surface.[14]

Layer V pyramidal cells are unique in that they mediate multiple pathways of perceptual feedback analysis.[14,15] For example, in the visual cortex layer V pyramidal cells are responsible for synchronizing corticothalamic activity with the thalamus via descending axons; they mediate feedback discrimination in columnar circuits via recurrent collaterals ascending through Layers I-IV; they mediate reciprocal interareal connections via laterally branching arboreal and basilar dendrites; and they mediate afferent cortico-cortical signal flow to the pre-frontal cortex (PFC) along both dorsal and ventral processing streams. Through lateral, vertical, elliptical, and recurrent feedback connections, layer V pyramidal cells bind multisensory frame data across the cortex with a functional refresh rate of roughly 15 to 30 frames-per-second (FPS), which means these neurons must process and neutralize incoming sensory spike trains at roughly every 30-60 milliseconds.[16] Loss of precise synchrony and coupling in these circuits would necessarily lead to loss of temporal fidelity in multisensory frame binding. Agonism, disinhibition, excitation, and nonlinear amplification in layer V recurrent circuits would necessarily lead to global multisensory frame aliasing errors, feedback synesthesia, and eventual perceptual overload.

Destabilization in thalamocortical feedback loops

The most potent psychedelics are $5\text{-}HT_{2A}$ receptor agonists; the highest density of $5\text{-}HT_{2A}$ receptors are in the dendrites of layer V pyramidal cells; layer V pyramidal cells bind information in feedback projections throughout the brain. Taking these factors into account it is reasonable to assume that psychedelic hallucinogenic activity is due to nonlinear signal destabilization and amplification via disinhibition recurrent layer V feedback projections. Psychedelic hallucination is achieved by partial or full agonism along recurrent layer V binding junctions; the introduction of a competing agonist in the $5\text{-}HT_{2A}$

modulatory system leads directly to loss of inhibition, under-constrained perception, and self-sustaining excitation in autonomic sensory processing circuits. Destabilization of layer V projections is most acute where signal travels in recurrent loops or feedback circuits that resolve and react to incoming sensory data in real time. The primary circuits for binding real-time sensation include the cortico-striato-thalamo-cortical (CSTC) loops, and the more distributed cortico-thalamo-cortical feedback loops (or thalamocortical loops) which pass information from the cortex either through the basal ganglia or directly back into the thalamus for discriminating and gating attention of incoming signal flow. These loops can be described as attention-controlled feedback filters which drive and stabilize external perception and behavior. CSTC loops provide real-time sensory feedback for fine-tuning eye movements, motor reflexes, emotional responses, and cognitive value placed on stimulus.[17] Destabilization in signal coupling along thalamocortical feedback pathways will necessarily lead to problems with sensory gating, multisensory frame resolution, working memory, and seamless temporal aliasing.

There are specific entopic perceptual effects one would expect to see as a result of instability in thalamocortical feedback loops between the thalamus to the visual cortex, such as a subtle flickering or pulsing of light intensity; geometric grids and matrices; the perception of halos or auras around light sources; increased luminosity of reflective objects; the softening of line and texture resolution; and the inability to hold sharp focal contrast between foreground and background in depth perception.[18] Sensory filling in the visual periphery relies on fast temporal aliasing of signal for motion detection, and this time-dependent temporal aliasing can be subverted by optical illusions which create a sense of movement in the periphery (Figs. 6,23). A competing 5-HT$_{2A}$ agonist would necessarily disrupt the precise inhibitory timing in the cortical columns needed for peripheral edge detection and sensory filling, leading to shifting line and depth ambiguities in the periphery along predictable pulse cycles. If the rate of multisensory frame saturation or neutralization was slowed or interrupted by even a few milliseconds, incoming sensation would begin to layer over itself with increasing levels of smoothing, liquidity, and phantom frame echo decaying in the wake of sensation.[19]

5-HT$_{2A}$ receptor agonists can destabilize multisensory perception in a number of ways. The most general explanation is that 5-HT$_{2A}$ agonists introduce a competing excitatory impulse that disrupts the precise timing of sensory binding in the apical dendrites and recurrent circuits of the thalamus and cortex. Evidence indicates that 5-HT$_{2A}$ agonists promote a late release of glutamate from layer V pyramidal cells following strong incoming spike trains, resulting in the generation of asynchronous excitatory postsynaptic currents (EPSCs).[1,11,12] Asynchronous EPSCs in recurrent sensory circuits are normally helpful for resolving important perceptual data, but if the subject is unable to inhibit evoked EPSCs caused by exogenous modulators (hallucinogens), this late signaling action can lead to glutamate flooding and tonic sensory saturation in perceptual neural assemblies, which is consistent with manic self-sustained states of hallucinogenesis.[20]

There is evidence that 5-HT$_{2A}$ agonists lead to lateral disinhibition in the cortex by blocking presynaptic uptake of 5-HT at the lateral inhibitory synapse, or by overriding tonic GABA$_B$ inhibitory postsynaptic potentials (IPSPs) with asynchronous EPSCs at the lateral-inhibitory synapse.[21,22] Loss of inhibition at the lateral synapses in columns of the visual cortex would lead directly to shifting and wiggling in peripheral line, texture, and contrast resolution. As thalamocortical feedback circuits become increasingly disinhibited, they may fall into coherent self-sustaining states of under-constrained perception,[23] promoting phantom sensory activity such as hallucination and spontaneous dream filling in the corners of the eyes. In the disinhibited or under-constrained psychedelic state, mild stimulus may not provoke hallucinogenic response, but intense stimulation would drive sudden localized feedback coherence, signal amplification, and resulting frame saturation and latency errors. The sudden shift from stabilized brain focus to states of elicited, recurrent thalamocortical feedback excitation can be described in terms of a nonlinear, non-equilibrium phase transition caused by energetic sensory drivers.[15]

5-HT$_{2A}$ cross-agonism and organism re-modulation

Looking beyond the cortex, it is worth mentioning that 5-HT$_{2A}$ receptors are also found in the midbrain, olfactory systems, the brainstem, intestines, and all over the body in smooth muscles and cardiovascular systems. There is some evidence that 5-HT$_2$ agonists have a secondary effect at the locus ceruleans in the brainstem (LC), promoting adrenal activity in the presence of strong sensory drivers.[1] Sensory driving of adrenal release may promote a synesthetic burst of emotional intensity accompanying any strong multisensory experience. There is evidence that 5-HT agonist hallucinogens inhibit sensory gating in the thalamus, allowing more raw sensation to flood the cortex;[17] this is consistent with decreased gating and nonlinear feedback amplification in thalamocortical loops. A common early side-effect of hallucinogen use is stomach tightening and intestinal cramping; this is undoubtedly due to 5-HT$_{2A}$ agonism interfering with modulation of smooth muscle contraction in the gut. 5-HT$_{2A}$ cross-agonism in the intestines can lead to nausea and purgation, and reports of intense hallucinations typically increase immediately following release of intestinal discomfort.[24] This indicates that radical interruption and re-modulation of all 5-HT$_{2A}$ pathways, from the intestines to the cortex, may be a common precursor to peak psychedelic experiences and states of intense bodily transcendence.

Because of the multiple systems affected by 5-HT$_{2A}$ receptor agonism, it would be overly reductive to point to a single pathway as being responsible for full psychedelic activation. The synergistic effect of multi-layered 5-HT$_{2A}$ agonism is felt subjectively as a throbbing or pulsation of energy which suffuses the entire body, builds in strength and complexity, and culminates in a cathartic multisensory release of highly charged transformative content. At the sensory level, glutamate flooding saturates perception. At the emotional level, adrenal response drives sensual intensity. At the frame level, aminergic interference leads to disorientation and loss of temporal ego cohesion. At the cognitive level, aminergic destabilization drives irrationality, depersonalization, and hallucinogenic dream states. At the circulatory level, 5-HT$_{2A}$ agonism promotes vasoconstriction and increases blood pressure. At the somatic level, an interruption of digestive functioning drives metabolic function and energetic intracellular signaling. At the organism level, the holistic effects of prolonged 5-HT$_{2A}$ agonism become nonlinear, meaning they feed back on themselves and begin to generate complex energetic output in response to sensory input over time. This multi-layered organism activation can be formally described as a runaway biological feedback process, or a nonlinear cellular signaling loop, which drives increasing cellular activity and complexity over the full duration of synergistic agonism.

Notes and References

1. Aghajanian GK, Marek GJ, "Serotonin and Hallucinogens". Neuropsychopharmacology. 1999 Aug;21(2 Suppl):16S-23S.

2. Ray TS, "Psychedelics and the Human Receptorome". PLoS One. 2010; 5(2): e9019.

3. Burnet PW, et al., "The distribution of 5-HT1A and 5-HT2A receptor mRNA in human brain". Brain Res. 1995 Apr 3;676(1):157-68.

4. Forutan F, Estalji S, Beu M, et al., "Distribution of 5HT2A receptors in the human brain: comparison of data in vivo and post mortem". Nuklearmedizin. 2002;41(4):197-201.

5. Pompeiano M, Palacios JM, Mengod G., "Distribution of the serotonin 5-HT2 receptor family mRNAs: comparison between 5-HT2A and 5-HT2C receptors". Brain Res Mol Brain Res. 1994 Apr;23(1-2):163-78.

6. WikiPedia.org, "5-HT2A Receptor". Internet Reference, 2010.

7. Azmitia EC, "Serotonin and brain: evolution, neuroplasticity, and homeostasis". Int Rev Neurobiol. 2007;77:31-56.

8. Nichols DE, "Hallucinogens". Pharmacology & Therapeutics Volume 101, Issue 2, February 2004, Pages 131-181.

9. Urban JD, et al., "Functional selectivity and classical concepts of quantitative pharmacology". J Pharmacol Exp Ther.;320(1):1-13. Epub 2006 Jun 27.

10. WikiPedia.org, "Protein kinase C". Internet Reference, 2010.

11. Aghajanian GK, Marek GJ, "Serotonin, via 5-HT2A receptors, increases EPSCs in layer V pyramidal cells of prefrontal cortex by an asynchronous mode of glutamate release". Brain Research V 825, 1-2, 17 April 1999, Pages 161-171.

12. Aghajanian GK, Marek GJ, "Serotonin Induces Excitatory Postsynaptic Potentials in Apical Dendrites of Neocortical Pyramidal Cells". Neuropharmacology Volume 36, Issues 4-5, 5 April 1997, Pages 589-599.

13. Spratling MW, "Cortical Region Interactions and the Functional Role of Apical Dendrites". Behavioral and Cog. Neuroscience Rev., 1-3 (2002) 219-228.

14. Jones EG, "Thalamic circuitry and thalamocortical synchrony". Philos Trans R Soc Lond B Biol Sci. 2002 Dec 29;357(1428):1659-73.

15. Lumer ED, Edelman GM, Tononi G, "Neural dynamics in a model of the thalamocortical system. II. The role of neural synchrony tested through perturbations of spike timing". Cereb Cortex. 1997 Apr-May;7(3):228-36.

16. See Chapter 05, "Limits of Human Perception".

17. Vollenweider FX, Geyer MA, "A systems model of altered consciousness: integrating natural and drug-induced psychoses". Brain Res Bull. 2001 Nov 15;56(5):495-507.

18. See Chapter 10, "Entopic Hallucination".

19. See Chapter 12, "Erratic Hallucination".

20. Geyer MA, Vollenweider FX, "Serotonin research: contributions to understanding psychoses". Trends Pharmacol Sci. 2008 Sep;29(9):445-53.

21. Kass L, Hartline PH, Adolph AR, "Presynaptic uptake blockade hypothesis for LSD action at the lateral inhibitory synapse in Limulus". The Journal of General Physiology, Vol 82, 245-267.

22. Shao Z, Burkhalter A, "Role of $GABA_B$ receptor-mediated inhibition in reciprocal interareal pathways of rat visual cortex". J Neurophysiol. 1999 Mar;81(3):1014-24.

23. Behrendt RP, "Hallucinations: synchronisation of thalamocortical gamma oscillations underconstrained by sensory input". Conscious Cogn. 2003 Sep;12(3):413-51.

24. Accounts of hallucinogens causing stomach unease and intestinal cramping taken from surveys of subjective reports.

25. Watts SW, "Activation of the mitogen-activated protein kinase pathway via the 5-HT2A receptor". Ann N Y Acad Sci. 1998 Dec 15;861:162-8.

26. WikiPedia.org, "Mitogen-activated protein kinase". Internet Ref., 2010.

27. See Chapter 13, "Psychedelic Neuroplasticity".

28. Belcheva MM, et al., "μ and κ Opioid Receptors Activate ERK/MAPK via Different Protein Kinase C Isoforms and Secondary Messengers in Astrocytes". J Biol Chem. 2005 July 29; 280(30): 27662–27669.

29. Bohn LM, "Mitogenic Signaling via Endogenous κ-Opioid Receptors in C6 Glioma Cells: Evidence for the Involvement of Protein Kinase C and the Mitogen-Activated Protein Kinase Signaling Cascade". J Neurochem. 2000 February; 74(2): 564–573.

30. Bruchas MR, et al., "Kappa Opioid Receptor Activation of p38 MAPK Is GRK3- and Arrestin-dependent in Neurons and Astrocytes". June 30, 2006 The Journal of Biological Chemistry, 281, 18081-18089.

Chapter 09

What is Nonlinear Hallucination?

Psychedelic Information Theory invokes nonlinearity to describe the perceptual effects of hallucination, but the term nonlinear has a variety of definitions which are sometimes confusing or unclear. To clarify the nonlinearity of psychedelic hallucination, the following is a description of formal nonlinear dynamics, broader definitions of nonlinear systems, and how each of these definitions may apply to psychedelic perception.

Nonlinear Systems

Nonlinear systems can be defined in terms of the complexity of output in proportion to input, also described in terms of sensitivity to initial conditions. The output of changes in a linear system are simple and can be modeled with a line on a graph. In contrast, the output of a nonlinear system feeds back on itself and becomes chaotic and complex; simple small changes in initial conditions will result in unpredictable and exponentially divergent data sets that cannot be easily predicted. In mathematical terms, the results of a nonlinear system begin to bifurcate, diverge, or split into multiple possible data points the farther out you attempt to resolve them. The results of a nonlinear system cannot be modeled with a linear function because linear functions plot sequential or additive complexity; nonlinear functions plot exponential or geometrically expanding complexity. The mathematical study of nonlinear systems has resulted in chaos theory, complexity theory, and the analysis of self-amplifying recursive systems such as fractals and cellular automata. Renderings of nonlinear systems output are considered to be of high intrinsic beauty, (Fig. 14)[1] and the repeating forms and patterns are often perceived as spiritual or mystical because they are isomorphic of chaotic or nonlinear systems in biology, nature, and the cosmos.

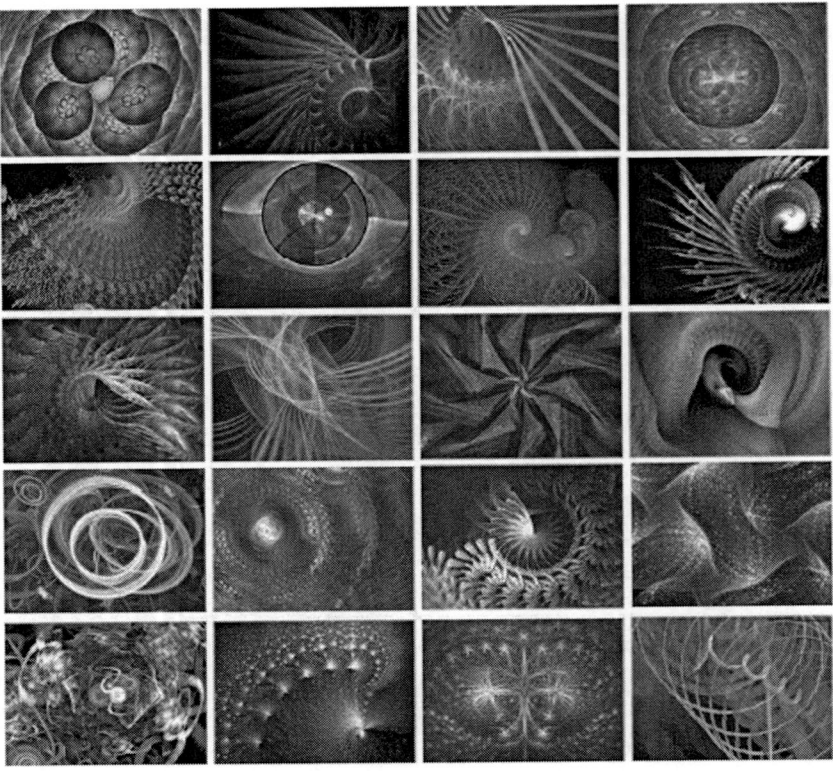

Figure 14. "Electric Sheep" fractals selected for an aesthetic voting experiment. Images chosen for intrinsic natural beauty. From Taylor, 2008.[1]

Nonlinear Consciousness

The physical world is a complex nonlinear system, but human consciousness perceives reality as a single linear sequential narrative that moves predictably forward in time. The linearity of perception is an indication that consciousness is producing stable, predictable output. If perception suddenly diverges into multiple unpredictable outputs for the same linear input, this is an indication that consciousness has destabilized and become nonlinear. A video feedback loop is an good example of a nonlinear perceptual system; each frame captures itself and the receding previous frame, and then itself and two receding frames, and then itself and three receding frames, and then itself and four receding frames, and so on, feeding back on itself at 30 frames per second until complexity recedes into chaos and infinity (Fig. 15). This is the mathematical definition of nonlinear system generating fractal complexity, or chaos, through an iterated map or recursive frame-stacking feedback loop.

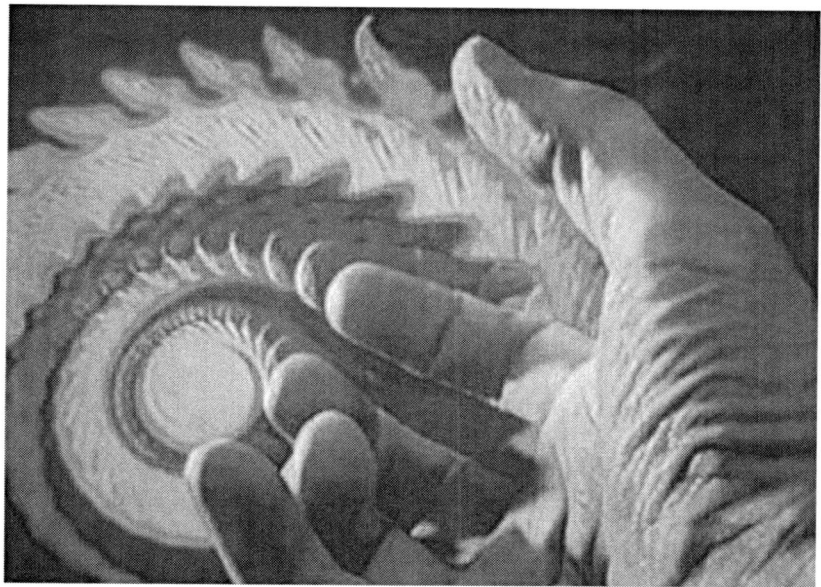

Figure 15. A video feedback loop creates a nonlinear system isomorphic of a fractal, where from recedes inward on itself, spiraling towards infinite complexity in under a second. From Hofstadter, 2007.[2]

Other examples of nonlinear consciousness may be less classically nonlinear, meaning not generating exponential complexity, but still lacking in linear formalism. For instance, consciousness may perceive itself to be in multiple places at once; it may perceive multiple data sets for the same input; it may see multiple different perspectives of the same scene; it may move sideways or backwards or completely outside of linear time. These would all be considered nonlinear perspectives of consciousness. Dreaming can be associatively nonlinear, which means narrative content moves unpredictably from state to state while retaining some tangential linearity. Psychedelics are famous for being progressively nonlinear, which means incoming sensation saturates perception and begins to stack over itself, generating increasing complexity of sensual intensity through time.

Phenomenology of Nonlinear Perspectives

By definition, a nonlinear system produces results with increasing complexity over time. In a linear perspective a human will parse a literal analysis of each object and then move on to the next object. In a nonlinear perspective the subject produces increasingly complex perceptual results for each object held in focus for the duration of that focus. For instance, a subject staring at a rock in a linear state may notice interesting shapes, textures, or colors; in a nonlinear state that same rock may provoke thoughts and visions of the birth of the universe and the origins of suns and planets and all solid matter leading up to the formation of that very rock. The linear perspective sees literal, formal attributes of the rock in the moment; the nonlinear perspective sees the rock as a temporary clump of energy bound in a cosmic information system receding forwards and backwards to the beginning and end of time. The metaphor of seeing the entire universe in a rock can also be applied to emotional epiphanies, autobiographical insights, passing fantasies, paranoid delusions, and so on. Whatever the focus of nonlinear perception, the object held in focus will be amplified with increasing salient complexity the longer it is held in focus.

The endless complexity of nonlinear perception can cause the subject to fall into perceptual loops which spiral, bifurcate, and recur with the formal qualities of a fractal (Figs. 1, 14). Frame information stacked in nonlinear psychedelic perception iterates on the order of 2 to 16 times a second, depending on drug and dose range, allowing for increasingly complex renderings of nonlinear information to the point of total sensory overload. Because of the quickly bifurcating complexity of nonlinear object analysis, the information produced in a nonlinear state emerges into consciousness much faster than information produced in a linear state. The production of fast, nonlinear data in the psychedelic state is often described as a download; an inconceivably large amount of information that compiles into memory almost instantly. The only way this amount of information can be processed through the brain is via nonlinear analysis; linear attempts to formalize psychedelic nonlinear information into words or pictures typically fall short of capturing the holistic perspective.

Nonlinear Hallucination

There are many colorful examples of nonlinear hallucination. Seeing geometric grids, webs, and spirals are nonlinear artifacts of destabilization of coupled oscillators in optic networks. Subjective reports indicate that DiPT produces unique nonlinear pitch transposition in audio networks, causing subjects to hear sounds modulated down an entire octave or more depending on the pitch and volume of stimulus. Auditory echoes, visual motion trails, and phantom tactile sensations are recursive artifacts of perceptual frame feedback. Perceiving multiple perspectives for the same input is a nonlinear bifurcation of multisensory coherence. Perceiving dream images superimposed over external space is nonlinear destabilization of visual memory recall. Seeing the formal boundaries of solid objects bend and melt into each other is a nonlinear destabilization of contrast and edge detection. Hearing a voice on the television or radio speaking directly to you is a nonlinear destabilization of semantic parsing and sequencing. Skipping time, missing time, or moving sideways or backwards in time is a nonlinear destabilization of temporal frame buffering. The basic tenet of psychedelic hallucination is that hallucinations move progressively from linear to nonlinear complexity depending on dose range and duration of effect; the higher the dose of the hallucinogen, the more disproportionately nonlinear, unpredictable, and complex perception will become in response to stimulus over time.

Notes and References

1. Taylor RP, Sprott JC., "Biophilic fractals and the visual journey of organic screen-savers". Nonlinear Dynamics Psychol Life Sci. 2008 Jan;12(1):117-29.
2. Hofstadter DR, "I am a Strange Loop". Basic Books, March 26, 2007.

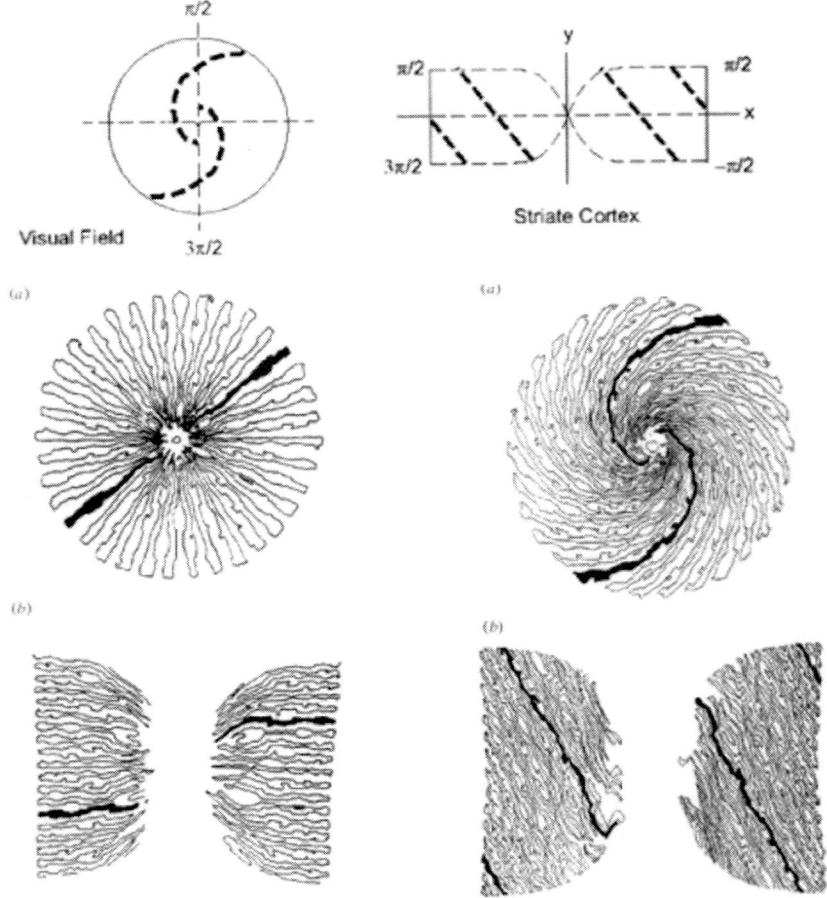

Figure 16. Spatial-relationship mapping between retinal cells with associated areas of the striate (visual) cortex. Images hitting the funnel and spiral ringed networks of the eye must be translated to lines and shades in the cortex for visual rendering. Geometric hallucinations, phosphenes, and entopic form constants arise from destabilization in (a) distance and (b) orientation selective retinal-cortical coupling. From Bressloff, 2002, Gutkin 2003.

Chapter 10

Entopic Hallucination

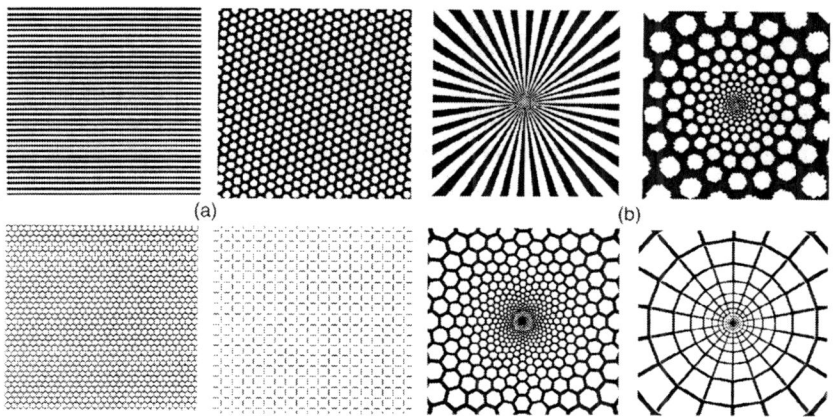

Figure 17. Geometric hallucinations, or flicker phosphenes, appear in form constants arising from destabilization in (a) distance and (b) orientation dependent retino-cortical signal coupling. From Bressloff, 2002., Gutkin 2003.

Entopic hallucinations, or phosphenes, are one of the most commonly reported visual effects of psychedelics. Phosphenes are a sensation of light caused by excitation of the retina by mechanical or electrical means. Pressure phosphenes can be created by applying pressure to the eyeballs through closed eyelids; flicker phosphenes are created in response to stroboscopic pulses of light; kinetic phosphenes are created in response to physical impact to the head, sometimes referred to as seeing stars. Entopic hallucinations are differentiated from eidetic or photographic hallucinations in that they originate within the neural connections between the eye and cortex (Fig. 16), as opposed to emerging within the cortex or midbrain. There is evidence that entopic phosphene patterns have influenced human cultural and religious archetypes since 10,000 BCE (Fig. 2).[1,2,17]

Entopic hallucinations fall into predictable geometric patterns and can be measured by formal properties such as form constant, flicker rate, rotation, drift, and decay. Common phosphene forms include web, grid, checkerboard, clover-leaf, honeycomb, spiral, funnel, or more amorphous floating blobs and stars (Fig. 17).[3] Phosphene patterns may match recurring patterns in the natural world, such as cells, stars, sand dunes, flowers, clouds, and snakeskin. Evidence suggests that the form constants of phosphenes are directly related to spatial relationships between the ring-like structure of the retinal cells and the grid-like or columnar neural structures of the visual cortex. The spontaneous production of geometric hallucinations is due to excitation and loss of stability in these retinal-cortical feedback coupling pathways. The transition from seamless visual aliasing to spontaneous geometric patterns can be described as a transcritical sensory bifurcation reflecting the spatial organization of the recurrent network.[4,5,6]

Pulses in the same frequency range as brain waves (theta to gamma) are most effective in producing flicker phosphenes.[3] Flicker phosphenes created by stroboscopic lights or mind-machines tend to be more amorphous at low frequencies(1-4hz), tend to fall into web, spiral, or cloverleaf patterns at medium frequencies (4-9hz), and tend to lock into grid, honeycomb, or checkerboard patterns at higher frequencies (9-16hz+). Flicker phosphenes will have slow lateral drift at lower frequencies; a rotational drift at medium frequencies; and will maintain stability or produce fast lateral drift at higher frequencies.[7] These phase-related transitions in standing wave shape are also seen in Chladni patterns created in vibrating plates (Fig. 31). Presumably any technology which uses pulsating frequencies to produce phosphenes, such as transcranial magnetic stimulation (TMS), must also use pulses corresponding to the frequency range of human temporal aliasing to produce substantially stabilized phosphene forms.[8]

Flicker Phosphenes and Hallucinogenic Interrupt

Taking what we know about the production of geometric hallucinations in response to pulse activity within specific frequency ranges, it is possible to extrapolate that the multisensory interrupt of any hallucinogen must fall into the same range of @5-40hz, which is the general frequency range of human consciousness, to produce phosphenes. According to the Control Interrupt Model of psychedelic action, any drug which produces a multisensory interrupt within the frequency band of waking consciousness will also necessarily produce flicker phosphenes and be considered hallucinogenic. If the multisensory interrupt is too slow or too fast, the drug may still be considered psychedelic, empathogenic, entactogenic, or dissociative, but it will be less likely produce significantly realized geometric flicker hallucinations. This same principle can be applied to audio and tactile sensory binding; any periodic interrupt within the frequency band of human sensory consciousness will necessarily induce field-like hallucinations with stable form constants and properties related directly to the interrupt frequency.

Figure 18. Examples of programmatic cellular automata. Repetition of simple algorithms create complex patterns of archetypal beauty. Levitated.net, 2010.

The evolution of flicker phosphenes can be described formally by the geometrical self-organizing feedback patterns seen in fractals (Figs. 1, 14), cellular automata (Fig. 18), or patterns arising from standing wave interference (Fig. 31). Under the influence of psychedelics, flicker phosphenes grow in intensity, become more elaborate, and become more structurally resolved over time.[3] It can be assumed that this is because the modulatory interrupt of a hallucinogen is being applied directly to the sensory binding pathways via pharmacological interaction as opposed to being applied to the retinal or cortical networks via external pulse stimulation. Because the modulatory interrupt of psychedelics is pharmacological, it is more difficult for the subject to fend off or ignore the interrupt to retain multisensory stability; the very pathways that maintain stability are the pathways which are being interrupted. In a very physical way, the modulatory interrupt of the hallucinogen is hijacking the sensory signaling pathways and overriding them with its own modulatory frequency. Because of this, the influence of the hallucinogenic flicker interrupt becomes explicit in sensory rendering; the subject may literally see or feel the pulsating geometric field interference as a fully embedded aspect of their perceptual reality.

Flicker phosphenes are the product of neurochemical saturation and have substantial signal decay. There is evidence that electrically stimulated phosphenes take as long as 10-15 seconds to fully fade once the periodic stimulus is removed.[9] Overlapping stereoscopic phosphenes will naturally create decaying interference patterns approaching fractal complexity. It can be assumed there is a saturation of signaling molecules that builds up at the site of synaptic interruption that persists for some period of time following each interrupt. The pulse of each interrupt can be described in terms of saturation attack and decay; the fade of each interrupt can be described in terms of saturation sustain and release (or ADSR envelope).[10] Full saturation would mean a complete white-out of sensory information at the interrupt site; zero saturation would mean the interrupt site is cleared of signaling molecules and is presenting a darkened resting state. Saturation at the interrupt site increases and decreases in intensity over the period of each interrupt; this change in chemical saturation over the duration of each interrupt is perceived as a flicker or pulse of sensory intensity.

Because a hallucinogenic interrupt pulses at many cycles per second, and because each pulse can have a saturation decay of many seconds, phosphenes will naturally drift laterally or radially across the visual field as they decay, creating overlapping webs of many arising and fading geometric patterns all visible within a single perceptual frame. This creates the formation of complex standing interference patterns. The web-like interference of multiple arising and decaying geometric grids creates a 3D meshwork that allows complex eidetic shapes to materialize spontaneously within the quickly morphing wire-frame (Fig. 20). Visual saturation is most intense at the interstices of the wire-frame mesh, creating the perception of bright dots or scintillating jewels where patterned lines overlap and intersect into nodes. These saturated pixel groups may correspond to actual hot-spots of neural activity saturating columns of the visual cortex. These hotspots are produced spontaneously in the wake of stimulus, creating a flood of glutamate wherever shafts of apical dendrites intersect with lateral projections from proximal neural columns.[18] Glutamate flooding at dendritic columns of pyramidal neurons is presumably the result of asynchronous glutamate release following 5-HT$_{2A}$ receptor agonism.[19]

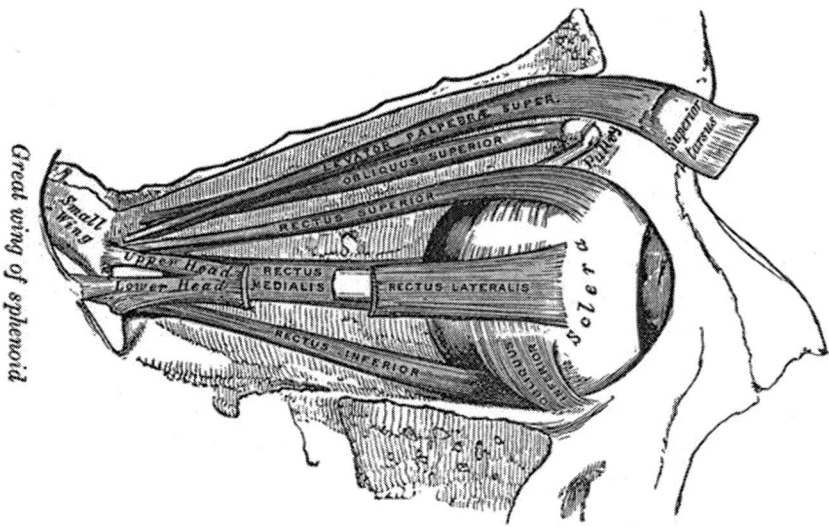

Figure 19. Muscles of the eye. Some subjects on psychedelics report pulses or rhythmic twitching in optic muscles that control focus, specifically the lateral rectus and inferior oblique. These pulses may generate pressure phosphenes related directly to frequency of pulsation. From Grey's Anatomy.

It is widely assumed that geometric hallucinations and flicker phosphenes originate between the optic track and cortex, but some subjective reports of psychedelic experimentation also describe a fast pulsation or rhythmic jitter felt in the muscles around the eyes. This sensation is most acute in the outside corner of the visual periphery, specifically along the lateral rectus and the junction where the inferior oblique passes over the inferior rectus (Fig. 19). This optical pulse may be difficult to discern in early parts of a psychedelic session, but becomes more acute and easier to sense as the session wears on. This rapid pulsation may be related to modulatory interrupt and saturation at the cortical columns that control optic muscles, generating a chain reaction in neural transduction felt as a muscle twitch or throb. Periodically interrupting the eye's finely timed saccades with a muscle twitch or pulsation may be enough to produce phosphenes.

Increasing or decreasing optic pressure naturally produces phosphenes; 5-HT$_{2A}$ agonism decreases ocular pressure. In his experiments with phosphenes in the mid 1800s, Johannes Purkinje applied an aqueous extract of belladonna (scopolamine, atropine) directly to his eye to produce phosphenes. Because the effect was localized, Purkinje proposed that phosphenes may be related to cycloplegia, or partial paralysis of the eye muscles.[20] Given these reports, it is reasonable to assume that any interruption of visual motor control, interruption of optic signal transduction, or change in optic pressure will produce phosphenes. Phosphenes generated by changes in ocular pressure or muscle twitch would be considered synesthetic representations of pressure waves rippling from intraocular fluid into receptive nerve junctions.

Entopic vs. Eidetic Hallucination

Geometric hallucinations, or phosphenes, are considered to be entopic, meaning they are a product of excitation and destabilization in spatial coupling between neural assemblies in the retina and visual cortex, and produce geometric patterns similar to wave interference patterns. Entopic hallucinations can be contrasted with eidetic hallucinations, which are more fully formed images that appear from visual memory or imagination. Psychedelic eidetic hallucinations are often more explicitly personal than the abstract geometric forms associated with flicker phosphenes. Over the course of a psychedelic session, hallucinations will start with flicker phosphenes and then increase in complexity from entopic to eidetic content, often containing a seamless mixture of the two. It can be assumed that eidetic hallucinations only begin once serotonergic modulation of the PFC has been sufficiently interrupted to allow cholinergic modulation of internalized mid-brain visualization to come to the fore.[11] The transition from entopic to eidetic hallucination is also associated with a transition from the high frequency beta or gamma state to a lower frequency alpha or theta state.

Meditation and auto-hypnotic exercises are targeted to produce states of hypnagogia associated with theta waves and entopic hallucination. Drugs which naturally drive theta waves in the brain are called hypnotics. Some psychedelics are naturally hypnotic, others are hypnotic only in sensory deprivation or under the influence of a theta-band periodic driver.[12] The hallucinogenic tea ayahuasca is a mixture of a high-frequency interrupt psychedelic (DMT) and a low-frequency hypnotic diver (the beta-carbolines harmine and harmaline, among others). This synergistic blend of high-beta interrupt and slow-theta attenuators means that ayahuasca should promote both fast beta geometric flicker phosphenes as well as slow eidetic theta dream snippets. This prediction can resolve paradoxical EEG analysis of subjects under the influence of ayahuasca, which sometimes indicates increased power in high frequency beta and gamma coherence,[13,14] but in the context of shamanic ritual shows increased power in slow-wave theta activity.[15]

Eidetic hallucination is considered to be rendered photographically or presented as a 3D virtual model. In psychedelic intoxication, a strange conversion of eidetic and entopic phenomena can occur when an eidetic image or symbol reproduces into a marching grid or kaleidoscopic network of repeating symbols with a juxtaposed eidetic image emerging within the repeating superstructure. For example, a subject may hallucinate a geometric grid of quickly spinning colored triangles, and as those triangles flicker across the visual field they suddenly cohere into a 3D wire-frame mesh of a more fully-realized eidetic snapshot of a human body or face. In addition to triangles, the overlaying grid may be composed of dots, circles, honeycomb, spiders, insects, centipedes, worms, snakes, reptiles, lizards, question marks, swastikas, teeth, piano keys, skulls, flowers, leaves, stars, eyes, billiard balls, dice, playing cards, human faces, alien faces, dancing elves, skeletons, clowns, jesters, writhing bodies, branching trees, cells, bacteria, paisleys, DNA, Japanese kanji, Byzantine tile patterns, Mesoamerican brick patterns, Native American totem patterns, Polynesian tiki patterns, and similar repeating archetypal forms.[16] The fast flicker rate and embedded kaleidoscopic nature of this type of compound hallucination often defies formal description or the ability to accurately capture in art or memory. The hallucinogenic perception of a complex embedded symbolic grid or kinetic fractal superstructure is unique to the psychedelic experience; it may be the visual essence of what makes an experience authentically psychedelic.

Notes and References

1. Williams JD, Dowson TA, et al. , "The Signs of All Times: Entoptic Phenomena in Upper Palaeolithic Art". Current Anthropology, Vol. 29, No. 2 (Apr., 1988), pp. 201-245.

2. Pettifor E, "Altered States: The Origin of Art in Entoptic Phenomena". Internet Reference, 1996.

3. Knoll M, Kuglerb J, et al., "Effects of Chemical Stimulation of Electrically-Induced Phosphenes on their Bandwidth, Shape, Number and Intensity". Sterotactic and Functional Neurosurgery, Vol. 23, No. 3, 1963.

4. Bressloff PC, et al., "What Geometric Visual Hallucinations Tell Us about the Visual Cortex". Neural Computation 14 (2002) 473–491.

5. Gutkin B, Pinto , Ermentrout B, "Mathematical Neuroscience: From Neurons to Circuits to Systems". Journal of Physiology, Paris 97 (2003) 209–219.

6. Ermentrout B, Cowen J, "A mathematical theory of visual hallucination patterns". Biological Cybernetics, 34-3 (1979) 137-150.

7. Observations on the correlation between flicker rate and the form constants and properties of phosphenes are based on subjective reports of stroboscopic light pulse machines.

8. Bokkon I, Kirby M, D'Angiulli A, "TMS, phosphenes and visual mental imagery: A mini-review and a theoretical framework". Symposium on Transcranial Magnetic Stimulation and Neuroimaging in Cognition and Behaviour Conference, Montreal, Quebec, Canada, 25 September 2008.

9. Dobelle WH, Mladejovsky HG, "Phosphenes produced by electrical stimulation of human occipital cortex, and their application to the development of a prosthesis for the blind". J Physiol. 1974 December; 243(2): 553–576.1.

10. See Chapter 06, "The Control Interrupt Model of Psychedelic Action".

11. Hobson, J. Allan, "The Dream Drugstore: Chemically Altered States of Consciousness". MIT Press, 2001.

12. Subjective reports show that some tryptamines, such a the psilocybin and psilocin found in magic mushrooms, naturally cause drowsiness even in loud sensory environments. Other tryptamines, like LSD, can have paradoxically trance-like or stimulant-like qualities depending on the environmental drivers of set and setting.

13. Riba J, Anderer P, et al., "Topographic pharmaco-EEG mapping of the effects of the South American psychoactive beverage ayahuasca in healthy volunteers". Br J Clin Pharmacol. 2002 June; 53(6): 613–628.

14. Stuckey DE, Lawson R, Luna LE, "EEG gamma coherence and other correlates of subjective reports during ayahuasca experiences". J Psychoactive Drugs. 2005 Jun;37(2):163-78.

15. Hoffmann, E, "Effects of a Psychedelic, Tropical Tea, Ayahuasca, on the Electroencephalographic (EEG) Activity of the Human Brain during a Shamanistic Ritual". MAPS Spring (2001) 25-30.

16. Accounts of geometric meshwork or marching rows of repeating archetypal forms are taken from subjective reports of psychedelic intoxication.

17. Nicholson PT, Firnhaber RP, "Autohypnotic Induction of Sleep Rhythms Generates Visions of Light with Form-constant Patterns". White Paper.

18. Nichols DE, "Hallucinogens". Pharmacology & Therapeutics Volume 101, Issue 2, February 2004, Pages 131-181.

19. Aghajanian GK, Marek GJ, "Serotonin Induces Excitatory Postsynaptic Potentials in Apical Dendrites of Neocortical Pyramidal Cells". Neuropharmacology Volume 36, Issues 4-5, 5 April 1997, Pages 589-599.

20. Melechi A, "Seeing Stars: The Shifting Geometry of Phosphenes". Trip Magazine, issue 10, 26-27, 2004.

21. Levitated.net, "Artifacts of Computation". Internet Reference, 2010.

Chapter 11

Eidetic Hallucination

Psychedelics can produce many types of hallucination, including geometric webs and grids;[1] distortions of space and time;[2] and photographic images of objects, people, or scenery. Hallucinations with a photographic, animated, or film-like clarity are called eidetic hallucinations, or eidetics for short. Eidetics share many of the formal qualities of dreams, visual memory, and imagination, and may be the most alluring aspect of experimenting with hallucinogens. Eidetic hallucinations rise and fall like dream snippets, rarely holding form for more than a few seconds before fading or shifting into another form. Eidetic objects, scenes, or people that become solid and retain their shape for an extended period of time are called frank or concrete hallucinations. Concrete hallucinations are often solid, immersive, indistinguishable from reality, and share many of the qualities of lucid dreaming, sleepwalking, and dementia.

The most commonly reported eidetic hallucinations seen on psychedelics are of people, faces, skulls, jaguars, snakes, plants, blooming flowers, spirits, aliens, insects, and other similar archetypes. Eidetic hallucinations can sometimes take the form of entire virtual worlds, spirit dimensions, invisible landscapes, and so on. Eidetics often emerge within a pre-existing entopic interference pattern that grows in intensity over time to produce more photographic or 3D rendered objects (Fig. 20).[1] Eidetics under the influence of psychedelics are most often reported with eyes closed or while sitting motionless in meditative trance. On high doses of psychedelics eidetic hallucinations may materialize with eyes open on any surface, pattern, or texture that's gazed at for more than a few seconds.[3]

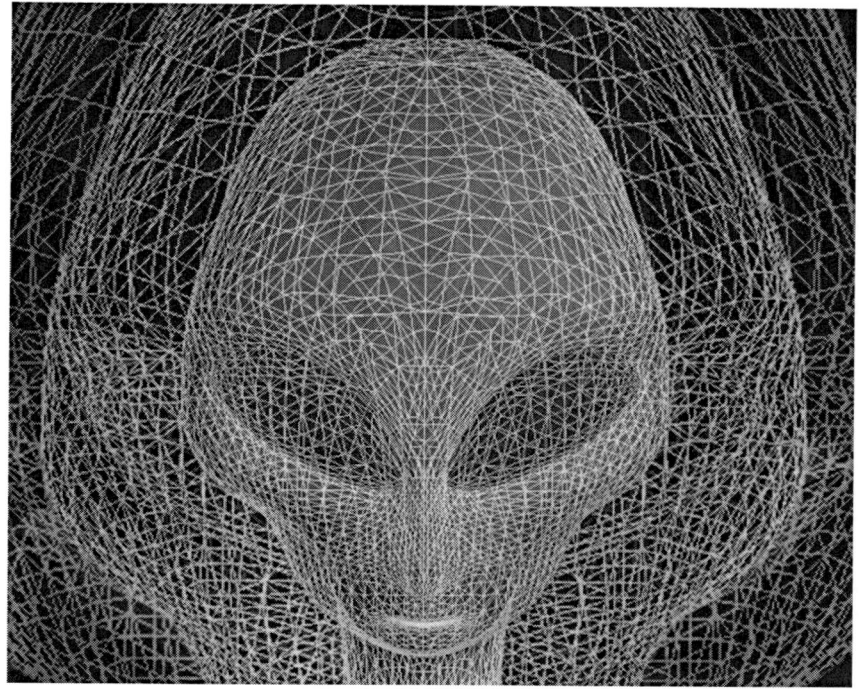

Figure 20. Eidetic tryptamine hallucinations, like this alien, typically emerge as snapshots or animations within a larger geometric interference pattern.

Psychedelic eidetics are progressive, which means they begin as non-durable form arising from patterns or noise, and then over a period of seconds drift, smooth, or lock into formal qualities which can be recognized as salient shapes. The process of smoothing or locking onto an eidetic form in a psychedelic hallucination requires some minimal amount of focus and concentration to sustain. The eidetic image may materialize, ooze, or pulse into clarity in response to the subject's concentration and focus, developing slowly like a Polaroid photo or film-reel fade-in. Losing concentration for an instant can cause the eidetic image to fade or shift into another image. Holding the eyes still will increase intensity of progressive eidetic imagery; blinking or flicking the eyes from side-to-side will wipe the visual memory buffer and cause eidetic images to fade; holding the eyes still again will cause previously held images to spontaneously rematerialize.[4]

$$H_3C\text{-}\underset{H_3C}{\overset{CH_3}{\underset{|}{N^+}}}\text{-}CH_2CH_2\text{-}O\text{-}C(=O)\text{-}CH_3$$

Acetylcholine

$$H_3C\text{-}\underset{H_3C}{\overset{CH_3}{\underset{|}{N^+}}}\text{-}CH_2CH_2\text{-}OH$$

Choline

Figure 21. Acetylcholine (ACh) modulates the medial-temporal lobe during memory storage, recall, and dreaming. Eidetic imagery in hallucination is associated with high ACh modulation.

The Hippocampus, ACh, Memory, and Dreaming

The processes of dreaming, memory storage, and memory recall are managed by the hippocampus.[5] The hippocampus receives perceptual information from the frontal cortex but is also wired tightly into the emotional limbic system and medial temporal lobe; which is why strong memories always have an emotional component.[6] Since the hippocampus is central in the formation, consolidation, and reconsolidation of all salient memory, we can also assume it is also the source of salient eidetic hallucination. The hippocampus is most active while awake and while dreaming. The process of moving from waking to sleeping is associated with a move from high beta or alpha activity down to slower theta and delta ranges. Deep sleep is associated with slow delta waves and low energy activation, while REM sleep and dreaming begin to produce beta activity and energy profiles similar to those seen in waking activity.[7]

Nocturnal dream activity is a process of memory consolidation.[8] In deep sleep and REM the stress chemical cortisol decreases communication between the hippocampus and neocortex,[9] and the process of REM and dreaming is stimulated by acetylcholine release.[10] Acetylcholine (ACh) is the primary messenger of the brain's cholinergic system, essential to hippocampal modulation of memory compression and recall (Fig. 21). Sleep-onset, sleeping, and dreaming are associated with an increase in ACh modulation of the brainstem and medial temporal lobe; this occurs along with a proportional decrease in serotonin, norepinephrine, and aminergic activity in the pre-frontal cortex (PFC). The interplay between these two systems acts like a tide between waking and sleeping worlds. Drugs which increase aminergic activity, such as antidepressants, should also decrease dreaming.[11] Similarly, the prolonged suppression of cholinergic activity and REM sleep due to deprivation or extended amphetamine use creates psychotic episodes which may be defined as bursts of dream activity erupting spontaneously into waking states.

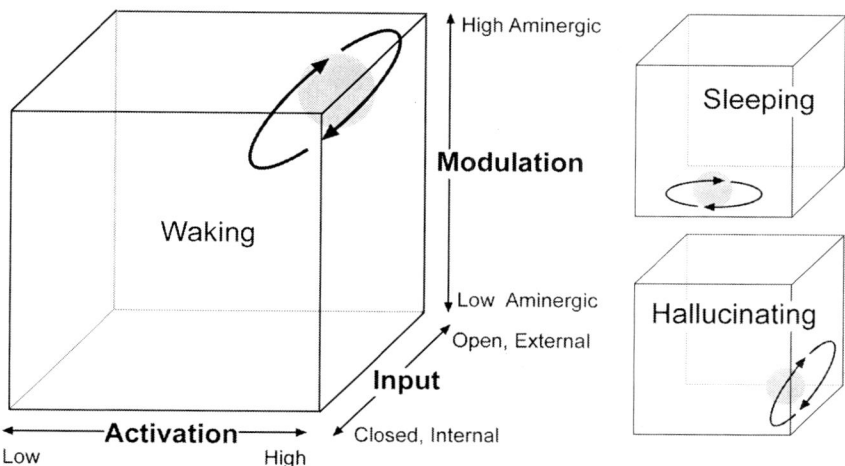

Figure 22. Hobson's AIM model shows patterns of (A)ctivation, (I)nput gating, and (M)odulation in various states of consciousness. Dreams and eidetic hallucination are associated with low aminergic and high cholinergic modulation.[11]

To describe the functional interplay between aminergic waking states and cholinergic dreaming states, J. Allen Hobson has proposed a three-dimensional AIM state-space model.[11] The interference between aminergic and cholinergic systems can be modeled by plotting the overall activation of the brain (A, high vs. low energy), the input of sensory signal (I, internal vs. external), and the signal modulation (M, aminergic vs. cholinergic). Using this AIM model we can present a snapshot of the waking, dreaming, or hallucinating brain in a graphic context (Fig. 22). A waking brain would be high in activity, input gated externally, with high aminergic modulation. A dreaming brain would also be high in activity, but input gated internally and high cholinergic modulation. Similarly, states of deep sleep, mania, and psychosis can also be described.

According to the AIM model, eidetic hallucination in a psychedelic session will not begin until external serotonergic modulation is sufficiently interrupted to allow internally gated cholinergic activity to rise to the fore of consciousness. Remaining motionless, closing the eyes, or sitting in a quiet darkened environment will stimulate the onset of eidetic hallucinations on psychedelics;[12] this is presumably because darkened stillness promotes sleep onset and an increase in internally gated cholinergic activity. The longer a subject under the influence of psychedelics remains motionless, the more photographically rendered the hallucinations will become. When the hallucinating subject rouses from trance and begins to move again, hallucination will lose photographic quality and return back to more generic entopic forms.

The ACh promotion of dreaming and REM has been demonstrated in animal research,[10] but only subjectively reported and presumed in humans.[22] Subjective reports of combining both the dissociative ketamine and the psychedelic LSD with pre-doses of galantamine and choline (both acetylcholine promoters) indicates that ACh promoters facilitate emotionally intense eidetic hallucinations, sometimes uncomfortable or unpleasant in nature, emerging beyond the subject's capacity to control.[13] This demonstrates that the production of eidetic imagery in response to ACh modulation is a spontaneous and automatic function of memory consolidation that cannot be easily controlled by the will or intent of the subject. The spontaneous production of salient eidetic memory makes psychedelics a useful tool in psychotherapy,[14] but the uncontrollable flood of eidetic imagery may not always be pleasant for the subject. States of intense eidetic hallucination may be associated with memory regression, imprinting, reconsolidation, and neuroplasticity.[15]

Anticholinergics, Concrete Hallucination, REM

Hallucinogens which target ACh receptors are reported to produce very vivid waking dreams and concrete hallucinations. Anticholinergics cause drowsiness, but at high doses also induce a disruptive sleep and a qualitatively unique form of delirium.[24] The commonly reported anticholinergic hallucinogens are the tropane deliriants atropine and scopolamine; found in deadly nightshade, belladonna, *datura*, Jimson weed, and members of the *Solanaceae* family.[16] Muscarine from the *Amanita muscaria* mushroom also interacts at the muscarine ACh receptors as an agonist. Tobacco also targets ACh receptors, but nicotinic ACh receptors instead of muscarinic receptors.[17] All plants and pharmaceuticals which target the cholinergic system are reported to be hallucinogenic at high enough doses. Cholinergic hallucinations are unique in that they may erupt into consciousness fully formed like dreams or fevered delusions.[18] In contrast, tryptamine psychedelics have progressive levels of entopic or erratic hallucination before reaching the level of concrete hallucination. Although *datura* and tobacco are common admixtures of traditional Amazonian ayahuasca preparations, experimentation with plants and drugs that target the cholinergic system at hallucinogenic doses is physically very uncomfortable and potentially lethal.[16,21]

Concrete hallucinations are similar to symptoms of dementia in that the subject literally cannot tell delusion from reality. Like a sleepwalker, the subject may think they are at the supermarket when they are actually looking into a closet. Psychedelics may produce this state of disorientation, but it is more commonly associated with dissociatives, deliriants, and pharmaceutical antihistamines or sleep aids. Suppression of REM sleep is associated with psychotic disorders,[23] and sleep deprivation for as few as three days can cause spontaneous periods of concrete hallucination and waking delusion.[19] Mixing anticholinergics with REM suppression can create highly realized waking lucid dreams and experiences of leaving the body and entering into parallel realities.[20] This indicates that periodic ACh REM consolidation of eidetic memory over the course of 24 hours is necessary for maintaining stability of consciousness. Activating eidetic memory consolidation with the use of psychedelics and extended REM trance-induction may be therapeutic for subjects suffering from depression, anxiety, or psychosis due to PTSD, insomnia, and other stress-related sleep disorders. Conversely, using psychedelics as stimulants to avoid sleep may lead to negative plasticity and persistent psychotic disorders.[15]

Notes and References

1. See Chapter 10, "Entopic Hallucination".

2. See Chapter 12, "Erratic Hallucination".

3. Content of eidetic psychedelic hallucinations taken from subjective reports and a survey of psychedelic literature.

4. Accounts of eidetic hallucinations arising progressively and being wiped from visual memory by eye movements taken from subjective reports.

5. LeDoux, Joseph, "Synaptic Self". Viking Penguin, NY, 2002.

6. LeDoux, Joseph, "The Emotional Brain". Simon & Schuster, NY, 1996.

7. Munglani R, Jones JG, "Sleep and General Anesthesia as Altered States of Consciousness". Journal of Psychopharmacology 6:399-409, 1992.

8. Stickgold R, Hobson JA, Fosse R, Fosse M, "Sleep, learning, and dreams: off-line memory reprocessing". Science. 2001 Nov 2;294(5544):1052-7.

9. Payne JD, Nadel L., "Sleep, dreams, and memory consolidation: the role of the stress hormone cortisol". Learn Mem. 2004 Nov-Dec;11(6):671-8.

10. Hobson JA, et al., "The neuropsychology of REM sleep dreaming". NeuroReport: 16 February 1998 - Volume 9 - Issue 3 - p R1-R14.

11. Hobson, J. Allan, "The Dream Drugstore: Chemically Altered States of Consciousness". MIT Press, 2001.

12. Accounts of psychedelic eidetic images becoming more intense with eyes held still, eye closed, or in a darkened room taken from subjective reports. Saccades, blinking, or any fast movement of the eyes wiping and refreshing visual memory also taken from subjective accounts.

13. Reported accounts of combining doses of both ketamine and LSD with pre-doses of 800mg of galantamine and 500mg choline report the eidetic visuals of these respective experiences as extremely intense, impossible to stop, and impossible to steer in a conscious direction. This experiments were conducted to enhance the capacity to remember the content generated in a psychedelic experience. Instead of aiding in memory imprinting, ACh modulation produced an opposite effect of visual memory flooding, creating a "Full-blown eyelid movie" that were not always pleasant and were impossible to control. Reports taken from personal e-mail correspondence with the test subject.

14. Grof, S, "LSD Psychotherapy". MAPS, 3rd Edition, 2001.

15. See Chapter 13, "Psychedelic Neuroplasticity".

16. Grinspoon L, Bakalar JB, "Psychedelic Drugs Reconsidered". The Lindesmith Center, 1997.

17. Cooper JR, Bloom FE, Roth RH, "The Biochemical Basis of Neuropharmacology". Oxford University Press, NY, 7th ed., 1996.

18. Accounts of experimentation with plant and pharmaceutical anticholinergics taken from subjective reports and a survey of literature.

19. Coren, S, "Sleep Deprivation, Psychosis and Mental Efficiency ". Psychiatric Times. Vol. 15 No. 3, 1998.

20. Zoe 7, "Into The Void". Worldwide Media, 2001.

21. Arnett AM, "Jimson Weed (Datura stramonium) Poisoning". Clinical Toxicology Review Dec 1995, Vol 18 (No 3).

22. LaBerge SP, "Substances that Enhance Recall and Lucidity During Dreaming". Patent Application number: 10/604,138; Publication number: US 2004/0266659 A1; Filing date: Jun 27, 2003

23. Cochen V, Arnulf I, Demeret S, et al., "Vivid dreams, hallucinations, psychosis and REM sleep in Guillain-Barré syndrome". Brain, ISSN 0006-8950. 2005, vol. 128 (11), pp. 2535-2545.

24. Itil TM, "Anticholinergic drug-induced sleep-like EEG pattern in man". Psychopharmacologia. 1969;14(5):383-93.

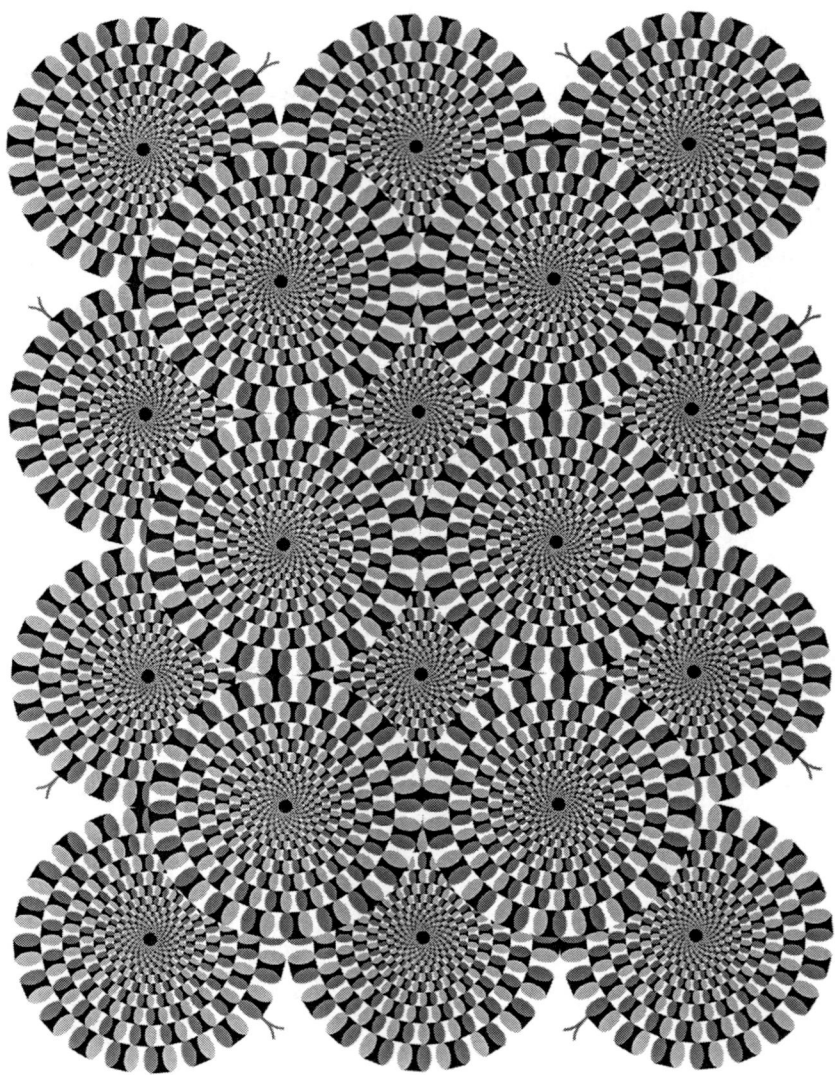

Figure 23. Akiyoshi Kitaoka's "Rotating Snakes" illusion. Stare at the center of any circle and the radial edges of nearby circles will appear to rotate. This image presents an example of the peripheral drift illusion due to contrast ambiguities in the visual field. This illusion exploits contrast expectations created by progressive 4-step gradients along radial tangents. The contrast expectations created by 4-step gradients are time-dependent and wired for motion detection in the periphery. The 4 degrees of color contrast around the periphery requires multiple frames to properly fill, creating a temporal ambiguity to edge aliasing exploited by this illusion. From Kitaoka, 2003.

Chapter 12

Erratic Hallucination

Hallucinations have formal properties that can shed light on their origins. Entopic hallucinations are characterized by geometric forms originating in the retina and optic tract.[1] Eidetic hallucinations are characterized by photographic images originating from the hippocampus and medial temporal lobe.[2] There is also a third type of hallucination not covered by these other formal categories; erratic hallucinations, or hallucinations originating in the loss of multisensory frame stability. Optical illusions that exploit rendering ambiguities in peripheral vision can be described as erratic hallucination. Tinnitus, or phantom ringing or buzzing in the ears can be described as erratic hallucination. Parasthesia, or phantom tingling sensations due to oxygen loss or nerve trauma can also be described as erratic hallucinations.

Like entopic hallucination, the origin of erratic hallucination is a destabilization of multisensory processing and sensory signal coupling. Erratic hallucinations caused by $5-HT_{2A}$ agonism include wiggling and drifting of line and shadow; frame stacking and recursive frame cascading; and temporal and spatial disorientation caused by loss of multisensory cohesion. Erratic psychedelic hallucination begins at low doses with simple formal boundary errors, and becomes more acute at higher doses, leading to the total loss of multisensory frame stability. Loss of multisensory frame stability under the influence of psychedelics resembles states of senility and schizophrenia.

Breathing Walls, Melting Textures, Creeping Carpets

Subjects under the influence of hallucinogens report breathing walls, creeping carpets, and melting textures. These effects are all similar in that they represent a loss of stability in sharp line, contrast, and texture detail in visual memory. This can be described as a rendering ambiguity error, and indicates a drifting of contrast information both laterally and radially across the cortex. This drifting in the visual field is most prominent in the periphery where the retinal blind-spots are working with incomplete data to begin with. This orientation ambiguity is exploited in optical-illusions which evoke rotational movement (Figs. 6, 23).

Hallucinations of creeping line, depth, and shadow are caused by a loss of lateral or localized inhibition within cortical circuits.[3] The level of disinhibition and drift in the visual field is presumably proportional to the dose of hallucinogen, and this assumption is proved correct by individual reports of hallucinogen use. While at lower doses there may only be a slight wiggling or drifting to the rendering of line and depth, at higher doses the lines and colors between solid forms may appear to bend, swirl, or melt into one another.[4] The inability to alias smooth lines or hold sharp contrast between objects is the definition of linear destabilization.

The melting or drifting of textures seen on psychedelics originates in the layers of the visual cortex, but there are other similar inhibitory mechanisms which stabilize sensory cohesion across the entire brain. By applying disinhibition to audio networks, a subject under the influence of psychedelics may hear an echo or murmur rising in the wake of each sound. By applying disinhibition to tactile networks the subject might feel phantom fluid sensations rippling along the skin. These hallucination patterns are distinct in that they arise like a wiggling or fluid ripple in the wake of stimulus, causing a loss of sensory field stability similar to a slow dripping or melting of contrast boundaries.

Frame Destabilization and Frame Stacking

The seamless nature of human perception depends on the fast updating of sensory frame information. Humans update waking frame information at roughly the beta range of consciousness, around 12-30 Hz, which is why animation, film, TV, and computer screens all appear seamless in the 24-60 Hz range. Psychedelics destabilize smooth frame aliasing by interrupting pathways responsible for multisensory binding.[5] At low doses hallucinogenic interruption is felt as entopic hallucination, but at higher doses modulatory interruption leads to more extreme frame destabilization. Subjects under the influence of tryptamine hallucinogens report sensory frame lag and slow-motion frames; frame delay or echo; frame flange or recursive looping; frame stacking or frame freezing; frame rewind and fast forward; dropped frames; split or bifurcating frames; frame skipping; and similar non-linear frame effects. These are all examples of extreme erratic hallucination linked to multisensory frame destabilization.

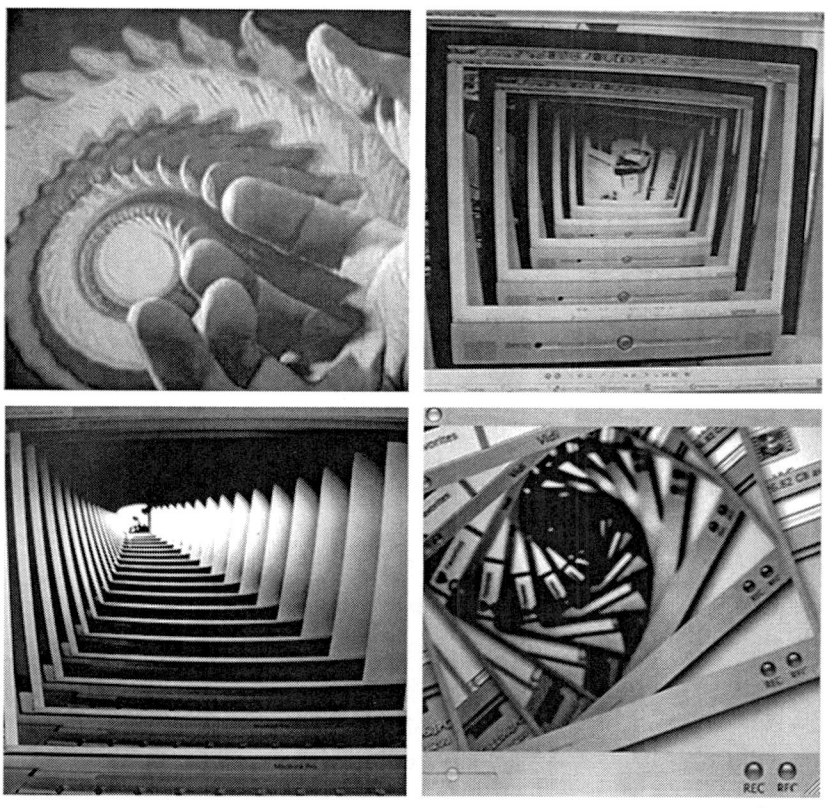

Figure 24. Examples of frame stacking caused by video feedback, which is isomorphic of fractal recursion, visual echo, and psychedelic hallucination. Frames stacked as few 16 layers deep quickly converge towards a vortex, a strange attractor, or a blur of infinite regression.

To account for various types of hallucination related to multisensory frame destabilization the following hallucinogenic Frame Stacking Model has been proposed.[6] To create the perception of fluid movement from frame to frame, any frame we perceive must be a composite of at least two frames, one arising and one fading. Each frame is associated with a neural spike train involving some feedback to the thalamus and basal forebrain to fix the frame's snapshot in working memory. These feedback circuits normally neutralize in about 1/15th of a second, allowing for multisensory frame update of @15 Hz. If hallucinogens interrupt the process of frame neutralization for some small period of time, each frame then begins to fade more slowly until frame data stacks up and feeds back on incoming perception (Fig. 24). As recurrent information from multiple receding frames replicates and stacks onto incoming frames, each perceptual frame splits or bifurcates in complexity. This iterating pattern of recursive complexity is the formal description of a nonlinear system.

Frame stacking is considered to be progressive with hallucinogenic dose and grows from mild to extreme. At low doses you might have four frames stacked in perception instead of two; three fading and one arising. With three fading frames you may begin to see softening of edges or intensification of colors as the saturation of each frame stacks over the next. With eight frames stacked you might see visual artifacts like jitters or trails in the wake of any movement, similar to visual flange or video feedback. While holding the eyes still, an increase in frame overlay makes solid objects crystallize into something very fascinating and precious, like a faceted jewel, creating a quality of temporal depth and luminance to surfaces and textures. An increase in frame overlay also creates enhanced edge smoothing between solid objects, which gives reality a sensation of liquidity or stretchiness like surreal art, graffiti, or a cartoon. As frames regress the perspective of perceptual space may begin to elongate like a fish-eye lens. If a fading frame produces an emotionally salient pattern, the salient layer can then feed back into the arising frame as a progressively animated eidetic loop. When sixteen frames are stacked in perception, the wake of overlapping and receding content causes frame overload, confusion, disorientation, dropped frames, ego loss, bodily transcendence, and missing time. Beyond sixteen stacked frames the information density becomes too large for the human brain to render; ego consciousness is overwhelmed and totally destabilizes into a swirling vortex of timeless transpersonal unity.

The Frame Stacking Model presumes that hallucinogens enable a perceptual frame buffer that allows for sorting and browsing through multiple simultaneous linear frames; or that frame perception might be splintered into a radial kaleidoscope of multi-threaded parallel processing frames. Within the context of frame stacking, psychedelic consciousness may enable the subject to scroll back and forth in time; retrieve multiple simultaneous memories from a single stimulus; and project multiple versions of the self into multiple imaginary future scenarios. If the consciousness of a single person can be momentarily realized within three frames – the arising frame, the fading frame, and a static frame which holds the idealized concept of self – then the persistence of six or more frames could lead to the fabrication of two or more fully realized identities within a single subject. This frame splitting effect may explain how people can have conversations with phantom friends or relatives, or how a shaman might invoke anthropomorphized plant spirits with distinct personalities.

Multisensory Destabilization and Schizophrenia

In large doses, hallucinogens can produce multisensory destabilization; a state where sensations, objects, time, and space become entirely decoupled from each other in consciousness. The sensation of time uncoupling or of space losing it boundaries is difficult to describe as hallucination, but it is clearly hallucination. Loss of sensory or temporal frame cohesion implies multisensory destabilization and erratic hallucination. Externally the subject may be awake and responsive, but internally the brain has lost all state data and is completely disoriented, much like acute senility.[7] This state can be simultaneously hysterical or terrifying, which describes the extreme mood shifts associated with transient schizophrenia. Schizophrenia is linked to the inability to retain multisensory frame stability and decreased ability to produce the fast gamma oscillations needed to focus and bind sensory perception.[8,9] Multisensory destabilization is also reproduced by the hallucinogenic dissociatives ketamine and dextromethorphan (DXM) by blocking associative NMDA pathways necessary for fast sensory binding.[10]

Notes and References

1. See Chapter 10, "Entopic Hallucination".

2. See Chapter 11, "Eidetic Hallucination".

3. Kass L, Hartline PH, Adolph AR, "Presynaptic uptake blockade hypothesis for LSD action at the lateral inhibitory synapse in Limulus". The Journal of General Physiology, Vol 82, 245-267.

4. Accounts of tryptamine psychedelics producing hallucinations of melting textures, creeping carpets, and breathing walls taken from a survey of subjective reports. Accounts of hallucinations of objects melting and pouring into one another taken from a survey of high-dose subjective reports.

5. See Chapter 06, "The Control Interrupt Model of Psychedelic Action".

6. The Frame Stacking Model of hallucination was proposed by a Canadian researcher who wishes to remain anonymous, and is presented here as a brief summary of a larger e-mail correspondence. The model is based on first-hand experimentation with LSD and *Salvia divinorum*, and has also been applied to hallucinations seen on DMT, psilocybin, 2-CB, N_2O, 5-MeO-DMT, Ketamine, DXM, and others.

7. Accounts of psychedelic intoxication matching states of schizophrenia taken from subjective reports and surveys of case studies.

8. Cho RY, Konecky RO, Carter CS, "Impairments in frontal cortical gamma synchrony and cognitive control in schizophrenia". Proc Natl Acad Sci U S A. 2006 Dec 26;103(52):19878-83. Epub 2006 Dec 14.

9. Colgin, Laura Lee, et al., "Frequency of gamma oscillations routes flow of information in the hippocampus". Nature 462, 353-357 (19 November 2009); doi:10.1038/nature08573

10. Bonta IL, "Schizophrenia, dissociative anaesthesia and near-death experience; three events meeting at the NMDA receptor". Med Hypotheses, 2004;62(1):23-8.

11. Kitaoka A, Ashida H, 2003 "Phenomenal characteristics of the peripheral drift illusion". Vision (Japan), 15 261-262.

Chapter 13

Psychedelic Neuroplasticity

Neural axons in the human brain are always branching and creating new synaptic connections to facilitate learning and development. Like the toning and bulking of muscle mass, neural connectivity, developmental growth, and plasticity are based partly on genetics and partly on the "use it or lose it" principle; the more you use a neural pathway the more robust and responsive it becomes, the less you use a pathway the weaker it becomes. Training and repetition build faster and more responsive connections; emotional attachments to concepts build more robust connections over time. The more a neuron or assembly of neurons is used in a specific exercise, the faster and more responsive those neurons will become when performing that task. This is how the brain learns new things and integrates new skills. Training, repetition, and reinforcement leads to long term changes in synaptic connectivity; these are the basics of neuroplasticity.[1]

Neuroplasticity is the physical mechanism which makes shamanism and psychedelic therapy viable. In dreaming, neuroplasticity is stimulated in response to daily routine and anxiety; in hypnosis neuroplasticity is stimulated in response to suggestion and reinforcement; in shamanism neuroplasticity is stimulated in response to dose, set, and setting. The efficacy of psychedelics in both shamanic transformation and clinical therapy relies on their unique ability to decouple the cortex, disassociate ego structures, and stimulate archetypal identity regression and personal transformation. No other class of drugs can claim to have such a radical effect on personality; radical personality change in response to brief psychedelic exposure implies neuroplasticity.

While there is no laboratory research to prove that psychedelics stimulate neuroplasticity, there is evidence that a single psychedelic session can produce long-term changes in personality.[2] People who take psychedelics sometimes adopt a new outlook on life, a new manner of dress, a new spirituality, perhaps even a new name to go with their new identity.[3] Self-reinvention is an integral part of psychedelic exploration and subculture. The forging of a new identity does not always happen in a single psychedelic session, but psychedelic experimentation can be a catalyst for sudden radical personality transformation. These basic observations make a case for psychedelics as facilitators of long term identity modification and neuroplasticity.

The Case for Psychedelic Neuroplasticity

Psychedelics can stimulate recall of lost memories and can also generate false memories; lost memory reconsolidation and false memory imprinting implies neuroplasticity. The brain builds tolerance to psychedelics quickly, but psychedelic tolerance can be surpassed by successively ingesting larger and larger doses.[4] Successive dosing and increasing levels of tolerance implies stress-based neuroplasticity. In the case of hallucinogen persisting perception disorder (HPPD), the subject retains some of the visual effects of hallucinogens long after the drug should have metabolized;[5] persisting reactions to neural stress imply neuroplasticity. Psychedelics have been used to facilitate cult induction and programming;[6] indoctrination implies identity-based neuroplasticity. Psychedelics induce peer and mate bonding in tribal subcultures; mate bonding implies identity-based neuroplasticity. Psychedelics can create positive long-term changes in mood and outlook;[2] long term outlook changes imply neuroplasticity. Finally, while lying in darkened silence, the psychedelic state resembles a deep dream-like trance; dreaming is known to facilitate memory compression and long-term memory potentiation (LTP).[7] Any drug which facilitates extended dream-like states should also facilitate memory compression, LTP, and neuroplasticity.

In programmatic terms, a psychedelic drug can be thought of as a back-door or reboot mechanism that allows the subject to enter a visually driven ego programming and debugging matrix; this state would be similar to hypnosis mixed with an element of lucid dreaming or creative visualization. To stretch the computer metaphor further, in the absence of hypnotic suggestion or shamanic control, the psychedelic debugging matrix will naturally drop into a maintenance mode where anxieties are brought to the fore like a screen-saver programmed to browse through repressed salient patterns arising within chaotic noise.[8] All of these programmatic metaphors for psychedelics are accurate, and all imply a spontaneous cataloging, compression, or re-organization of existing synaptic memory via nonlinear eidetic emotional cues; this implies synaptic testing and strengthening in response to pre-existing anxiety, which implies neuroplasticity.

Physiology of Psychedelic Neuroplasticity

Hallucinogens which target the 5-HT_{2A} receptor can influence cellular functioning via the activation of G-proteins and intracellular secondary messengers. The signaling pathways mediated by the 5-HT_{2A} receptor include the activation of PKC and MAPK, protein kinases which energize enzymes to perform complex cellular maintenance. The activation of PKC undoubtedly plays a role in the production and maintenance of long term memory. Evidence shows that inhibiting PKC activation in the cortex for as little as a few hours can cause the rapid erasure of long-term memory associations.[11] It is obvious that PKC is a fundamental part of memory formation and retention, and it is reasonable to assume that drugs which stimulate PKC activity may enhance or alter the processes of memory formation, recall, retention, and plasticity.

The process by which PKC mediates memory associations is still unknown, but the primary assumption is that PKC interacts with diglycerides (DAG) at the intracellular membrane to mark energetic signaling areas for receptor formation and synaptic strengthening. The secondary signaling cascade goes like this: The 5-HT_{2A} receptor is stimulated with an agonist, activating phospholipase C (PLC) in the cell membrane, which then chops a phospholipid (PIP_2 or PI) at the membrane into an IP_3 group and DAG. The DAG stays near the membrane while IP$_3$ activates the release of calcium (Ca^{2+}) from the endoplasmic reticulum, which then activates PKC, which allows PKC to carry energy back to the cell membrane near the DAG site before activating other enzymes and intracellular substrates. PKC performs its job by moving phosphate groups around the cytoplasm and activating cellular enzymes such as adenosine which forms AMP, ADP, and ATP by linking with phosphate groups in chains of up to three at once, allowing metabolic energy to move quickly to other sites throughout the cell. The addition and removal of phosphates to and from proteins is a fundamental part of all organic metabolic processes; 5-HT$_{2A}$ agonists stimulate this phosphorylation process through PLC, IP$_3$, Ca^{2+}, and subsequent PKC activation.

The fact that 5-HT$_{2A}$ agonists stimulate PKC and fundamental metabolic processes indicates a strong case for psychedelic neuroplasticity. It is interesting to note that Salvinorin A, from *Salvia divinorum*, also activates these same phosphorylation pathways through the G-coupled kappa-Opiod receptor.[12] It is also interesting to note that of all the hallucinogenic compounds that occur in nature, psilocybin (found in magic mushrooms) is the only one that comes with its own phosphate group (which is stripped to make psilocin), and also appears to be the weakest tryptamine agonist at the 5-HT$_{2A}$ receptor.[13] While it is tempting to assert that PKC phosporylation is at the root of all hallucinogenesis and psychedelic effect, it has been demonstrated that 5-HT$_{2A}$ mediated PI hydrolosis is not always a good indicator of psychedelic potency.[14] Although there are multiple factors responsible for hallucinogenesis, psychedelic stimulation of PKC activity undoubtedly plays a role in perturbing and stimulating persistent memory functions and promoting potential potent neuroplasticity.

Other research indicates that LSD activates cellular mechanisms to promote expression of genes responsible for encoding c-Fos and Arc proteins, particularly in the pre-frontal cortex (PFC).[15] c-Fos is essential to cell proliferation, differentiation, and cellular defense, while Arc (activity-regulated cytoskeleton-associated protein) regulates the formation and repair of the scaffolding maintaining neural shape and stability. By activating expression of c-Fos and Arc proteins in PFC neurons, LSD may promote potent neuroplasticity, cell proliferation, cell repair, and synaptic generation in neurons responsible for identity. Presumably any selective 5-HT$_{2A}$ agonist will produce similar results, making hallucinogenic tryptamines primary candidates for cellular signal strengthening and profound identity-based neuroplasticity.

Positive and Negative Plasticity

Shamanic transformation may stimulate neuroplasticity by helping the subject realize a more transcendent or spiritually integrated vision of themselves. The logic follows that visualization of a transcendent inner self will reinforce positive personality traits and behavioral changes to synchronize with inner idealization. Shamanic identity transformation is not instantaneous, but instead follows an integrative process of synaptic testing and reinforcement over a period of days to weeks. Some psychedelic therapy stimulates neuroplasticity using techniques similar to the ten-step program employed by Alcoholics Anonymous (AA), where the subject takes a clinical inventory of their life and behaviors and assesses each area where they need forgive, accept, or make changes. In psychedelic therapy the process of uncovering and severing negative pathways is called catharsis; the process of wiring and reinforcing new pathways is called integration. These are examples of positive psychedelic plasticity used to maximize positive social integration. These processes are sometimes slow and require some small amount of mental discipline and behavioral follow-through for success.

There are many examples of negative psychedelic neuroplasticity. Renegade schools of ayahuasca sorcery and witchcraft employ some of the most elaborate and lethal mind-games ever devised, including the constant fear of attack by rival sorcerers through poisons, curses, dream invasion, and magical darts that may induce paralysis, cancer, death, or insanity.[9] The traditional shaman's constant stress of exposure to the effects of black magic mirrors paranoid psychosis and post-traumatic stress disorder; this implies negative plasticity. Exposing any subject to extended and repeated psychedelic sessions may force stress-driven plasticity associated with PTSD, torture, isolation, and sensory deprivation. Psychedelics may speed techniques of ego deprogramming and imprinting associated with brainwashing or cult indoctrination;[6] this implies mind control and negative neuroplasticity. Psychedelics may produce psychotic breaks where subjects become violent and deranged, or may reinforce delusional, messianic, paranoid, sociopathic, antisocial and megalomaniacal identity traits;[10] this also implies negative neuroplasticity. Thus, forging new synaptic pathways to radically alter identity structures is not always a good thing, this process can induce pathology as easily as it can reduce pathology.

Tribal Imprinting and Viral Neuroplasticity

One of the most interesting aspects of psychedelics is that group psychedelic experimentation can catalyze spontaneous organization of tribal subcultures and grassroots political movements. According to PIT, if you destabilize the top-down regulating influence of culture over a small group of peers, energetic tribal organizations will spontaneously emerge within those groups; this is an extrapolation of control theory and tenets of distributed cognition. Modern history has demonstrated that if you sprinkle LSD or psychedelic mushrooms over a major city, then flower children will blossom and form drum circles and begin to reproduce. But close observation of modern psychedelic subcultures reveals that radical identity reinvention is not a function of spiritual freedom or political subversion, but is more a viral form of tribal bonding and indoctrination. For example, the hippies of 1960s and the ravers of 1990s each preached freedom and individuality, yet each culture had strictly controlled tribal uniforms, politics, musical styles, and rituals, and ostracized outsiders as being squares or un-hip. This indicates that psychedelic tribal organization and identity reinvention is not a linear function of freedom of expression or social liberation, but is instead a nonlinear amplification of the typical motivators of social elitism, the fears of being ostracized, and the reinforcements of tribal acceptance; all of which strongly affect identity-based neuroplasticity. Presumably any tribe, cultural group, religion, cult, or government can employ psychedelic neuroplasticity to similar social organizing effect.

Notes and References

1. LeDoux, Joseph, "Synaptic Self". Viking Penguin, NY, 2002.

2. Griffiths, R.R., "Psilocybin can occasion mystical-type experiences having substantial and sustained personal meaning and spiritual significance". Psychopharmacology (2006) 187:268–283.

3. Observations of individuals adopting new names and new identities in response to psychedelic indoctrination come from subjective reports and first-hand observations of psychedelic subcultures.

4. Gresch PJ, Smith RL, Barrett RJ, Sanders-Bush E., "Behavioral tolerance to lysergic acid diethylamide is associated with reduced serotonin-2A receptor signaling in rat cortex.". Neuropsychopharmacology. 2005 Sep;30(9):1693-702.

5. Abraham HD, Duffy FH, "EEG coherence in post-LSD visual hallucinations". Psychiatry Res. 2001 Oct 1;107(3):151-63.

6. Groups linked to the weaponized use of psychedelics include the Manson Family, the SLA, Aum Shinrikyo, the CIA, and the United States Department of Defense.

7. Hobson, J. Allan, "The Dream Drugstore: Chemically Altered States of Consciousness". MIT Press, 2001.

8. Accounts of psychedelics producing a screen saver or hypnotic autopilot of unresolved anxieties and salient attractors are taken from subjective reports and surveys of psychedelic literature.

9. Beyer, SV, "Singing to the Plants: A Guide to Mestizo Shamanism in the Upper Amazon". University of New Mexico Press (October 31, 2009).

10. Reports of psychedelics facilitating symptoms of persistent psychosis taken from subjective reports and a survey of psychedelic overdose case studies.

11. Shema R, Sacktor TC, Dudai Y, "Rapid erasure of long-term memory associations in the cortex by an inhibitor of PKM zeta". Science. 2007 Aug 17;317(5840):951-3.

12. Bohn LM, "Mitogenic Signaling via Endogenous κ-Opioid Receptors in C6 Glioma Cells: Evidence for the Involvement of Protein Kinase C and the Mitogen-Activated Protein Kinase Signaling Cascade". J Neurochem. 2000 February; 74(2): 564–573.

13. Ray TS, "Psychedelics and the Human Receptorome". PLoS One. 2010; 5(2): e9019.

14. Nichols DE, "Hallucinogens". Pharmacology & Therapeutics Volume 101, Issue 2, February 2004, Pages 131-181.

15. Nichols CD, Sanders-Bush E, "A Single Dose of Lysergic Acid Diethylamide Influences Gene Expression Patterns within the Mammalian Brain". Neuropsychopharmacology (2002) 26 634-642.

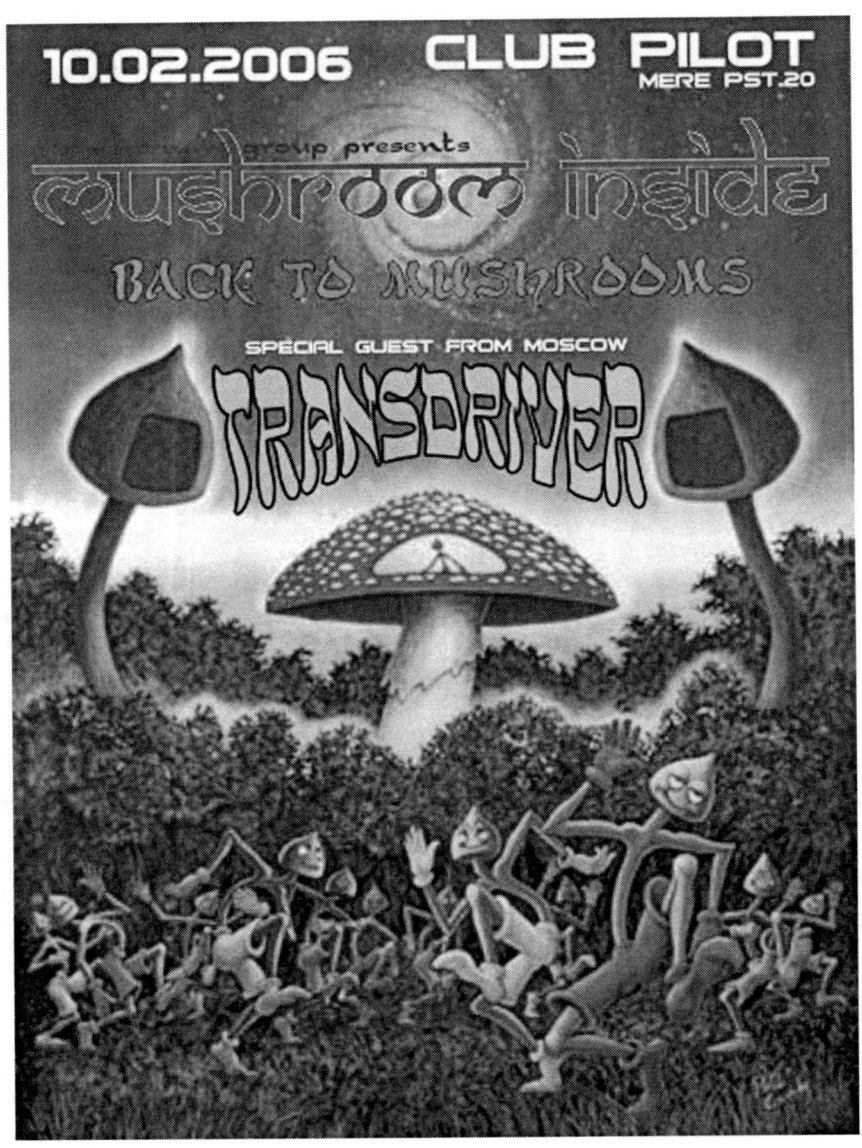

Figure 25. Flyer for a 21st century mushroom trance party entitled, "Mushroom Inside: Back to Mushrooms," where a DJ inside a giant amanita mushroom controls a synchronized crowd of psilocybe-headed dancers through giant amplifiers made of psilocybin mushrooms. Like marionettes, the dancers assume archetypal forms of resonating Chladni patterns or fractal plane-filling curves in audio-motor synesthesia with the music. Note the ecological overtones as the grass, trees, and galaxy keep tempo with glowing approval.

Part II

Shamanism in the Age of Reason

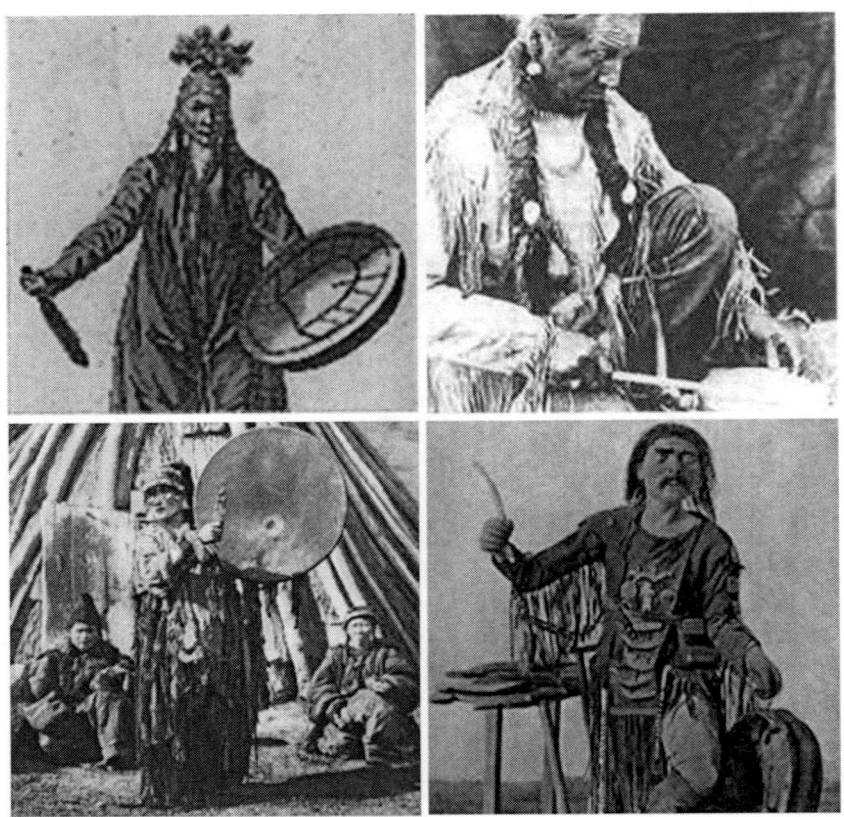

Figure 26. Pictures of the shaman from four different traditions. Clockwise from top: Tartar, Native American, Siberian, and Yakut. All shamen use medicine drums to control the tempo and amplitude of energy oscillating through the sacred circle.

Chapter 14

What is Shamanism?

The origins of shamanism are rooted in spirituality and myth, but the power of shamanism is entirely real. It is the goal of this text to explore rational limits and applications of shamanic power beyond the paradigms of mythology and faith healing. The subtitle of this text is "Shamanism in the Age of Reason," so it seems fitting to provide a good definition for shamanism. There are many definitions that have something to do with tribal healers, witch doctors, ritual plant magic, and/or dealing with the spirit world; these definitions conjure images of pre-industrial folk medicine steeped in superstition. Relegating shamanism to the bin of folk medicine fails to account for the sophistication of shamanic tradecraft, methodology, or the varying levels of shamanic manipulation. Traditional shamanism may be cloaked in the veil of superstition, but behind the veil is the real science of programming human belief and behavior with a blend of mysticism, ritual, and hallucinogenic drugs.

Instead of focusing on the many societal roles and functions a shaman might fill, PIT takes a broader view and starts with this definition: Shamanism is the craft of evoking spontaneous organization of psychedelic information in a subject or group of subjects to promote plasticity, imprinting, and transformation. Psychedelic information implies holistic or meta level manipulation of memory and identity, and this definition fulfills the functions of therapy, sorcery, mind control, applied psychedelic science, targeted neuroplasticity, behavioral conditioning, and tribal bonding. The technology of evoking and imprinting psychedelic information is inherently neutral; the shaman learns to apply this technology for healing and positive plasticity, the sorcerer succumbs to the temptation to use this technology for black magic and negative plasticity.

Transformational Plasticity and Imprinting

The power of shamanism can be measured by the shamanic ability to transform subjective beliefs and behaviors. A shaman can transform the subject in the literal sense, through diet and chemical manipulation; or in the figurative sense, by altering the subject's paradigm and perception of reality. Both of these transformations imply targeted neuroplasticity. The extreme diets and psychedelic medicine catalyze spontaneous stress-based reorganization of neural identity structures, and the shamanic mythology creates the semantic frame through which the subject parses the transformational experience. Although psychedelics have been tested in brainwashing and hostile interrogation, the process of psychedelic imprinting usually works best if the subject is ready and willing to receive the transformation.[1]

Some aspects of psychedelic imprinting are automatic and spontaneously generated like dreams;[2] in this case the shaman's job is to apply the medicine and essentially look important doing nothing. In other instances the subject may have an adverse reaction to the medicine, or become lost in the psychedelic space; in this case the shaman may intervene with a spirit song, a meditative chant, or a rhythmic breathing exercise to guide the subject through the transition. In traditional or loosely organized shamanic ceremonies, the level of intervention and depth of psychedelic imprinting is controlled by ritual, shamanic intent, and group intuition; in clinical psychedelic therapy the depth of psychedelic imprinting is controlled by protocol.

Shamanic Reputation and Expectant Plasticity

If a shaman gains a reputation for being transformative, subjects will seek them out expecting to be transformed. Similarly, a popular shaman may become the target of a rival shaman seeking to curse them or bring them down with magic darts. Both scenarios indicate that the shaman has successfully imprinted his own supernatural abilities to the point of viral plasticity. A shaman does not need psychedelic drugs to accomplish this, any guru with a transformational philosophy and self-promotional streak can achieve this level of influence. The shaman differs from the New Age guru only by having mastery of the plants and the spirit world, which is rudimentary psychopharmacology and ritual transcendence. By offering his or her self as the path to sacred wisdom or healing, or by telling tales of supernatural battles with other sorcerers, the shaman implies that he or she is more powerful than the medicine they employ. Shamanic reputation builds subjective expectations, and in many ways is a very clever set-up and misdirection similar to priming a magic trick or a placebo. If the subject already believes the shaman has supernatural power, the task of transforming them with the medicine is the easy part.

By crafting a supernatural reputation, the shaman starts the process of bending the subject's beliefs and expectations long before the medicine is applied. In hostile interrogation and indoctrination techniques, this process of bending subjective beliefs is called "softening up" the subject, or priming neuroplasticity to be vulnerable to imprinting. If the subject does not appear to respect the shaman's supernatural authority, the shaman may become withholding and demand that the subject follow certain strange rules before applying the medicine. Establishing authority, submissiveness, and strictly enforced rules gives the shaman implicit control over the subject, and sets the stage for applying transformation. Even if the subject does not believe the shaman's mythology, by forcing the subject to follow ritual protocol the shaman establishes the power dynamic necessary for controlling the ceremony and imprinting the subject.

Shamanism, Chaos Magic, and Belief as Toolkit

The shaman's role will always be intertwined with the spiritual belief of the larger tribe or culture. The mythology is not important, a good shaman can adapt any mythology or belief to transformational ritual. Instead of preaching the mythology, the shaman exploits the mythology as a handle or tool for interfacing with and manipulating the subject's core identity structures. By adopting a mythology that's alluring to the patient, the shaman can apply identity transformation within a seamless spiritual context. The process of finding or seeding an emotional handle is a skill that can be learned, but it can also be purely intuitive. The technologies of religion, propaganda, agitprop, and social activism all use negative emotional handles to influence people's beliefs and behaviors; shamanism employs many of the same techniques with positive emotional handles. The practice of manipulating belief like a tool to produce transformative results has become popularly known as chaos magic.[3]

The bulk of available literature on shamanism focuses on sprits, spirit mythology, and the ways in which the shaman communes with plant and spirits to gain supernatural insights. The allure and power of a drug that allows the user to talk directly with spirits is obvious, but fascination with spirits and transcendence may also be a handle used by the shaman to manipulate and imprint a willing subject. Western spiritual seekers are quickly enamored with the romanticism of entheogenic spirit communion, this is not something a good shaman would overlook; this is something that can be easily exploited. Whether the subject comes looking for Jesus, God, plant spirits, healing, or transcendence, the spiritual passions of the subject are the most powerful items in the shaman's entire toolkit.

Shamanic Practice and Seeking Balance

The role of the shaman has always been to apply transformation, typically to restore balance and harmony within tribal units. The shaman works by organizing the flow of energy and information within individuals and tribal structures. The shaman synergizes many layers of transformation in the act of brewing and ingesting psychoactive sacraments, and uses mythology and sacred ritual to facilitate communication, navigate conflict, and fine-tune the overall health of the tribe. Since shamanic transformation can be used for both healing and sorcery, it is logical that the larger tribe will only tolerate such power as long as it is more therapeutic than destructive. Because of this dynamic, a practicing shaman may be inherently distrusted, and will always walk the line between outcast and savior. The romantic character of shamanism relies heavily on this outcast trope. If the shaman fails at the basic tasks of healing and conflict resolution, or abuses shamanic technology to undermine the well-being of the tribe for personal gain, then the shaman loses power and risks being ostracized by the tribe. Thus, the shaman's power is limited and ultimately defined by the trust placed in him by the larger tribe.

Notes and References

1. Groups linked to the weaponized use of psychedelics include the Manson Family, the SLA, Aum Shinrikyo, the CIA, and the United States Department of Defense.

2. See Chapter 13, "Psychedelic Neuroplasticity".

3. WikiPedia.org, "Chaos Magic". Internet Reference, 2010.

Chapter 15

An Overview of Physical Shamanism

Physical Shamanism, or Shamanism in the Age of Reason, is differentiated from Spiritual Shamanism in that physical shamanism relies on models of neural oscillators and resonant wave entrainment as opposed to spirit models of channeling, telepathy, or clairvoyance. The Control Interrupt Model presents a description of physical shamanism based on the precision coupling of a multisensory hallucinogenic interrupt to a resonant environmental driver.[1] Physical shamanism assumes the human brain in a destabilized state acts as a resonant oscillator, or a nonlinear information processing system; thus shamanism can be defined as the application of resonant drivers to mediate complex phase transitions between multi-stable states of consciousness.[10,11] The techniques of physical shamanism are often used in concert with a hallucinogen in order to entrance or hypnotize a subject or group of subjects into a targeted mystical state.

Spirit Voices, Shamanic Songs, and Strange Attractors

When a shaman takes a psychedelic he or she hears the spirit voices and intuitively learns to sing the spirit songs. These songs are taken directly from the shaman's head as the psychedelic begins to interrupt consciousness. In many ways these sacred songs, or *icaros*, are attempts to recreate the voice and tone of the pharmacological interaction at various stages of the psychedelic experience. The voice of the shamanic medicine is not human in the typical sense, the psychedelic voice is described more in terms of the repetitive bleeping and blooping of machine code; a biological thrumming; an electronic or alien pulsation; a guttural river of slurping and squelching sounds; the great wheeze of a mystical reed organ; the chirping of crickets; the croaking of frogs; or the fast-clicking communication of an insect intelligence.[2,3] All of these colorful metaphors are the same in that they perfectly describe a resonant standing wave in the alpha to gamma range driving amplitude along multisensory perceptual bands. As the hallucinogenic voice grows in strength, the resonance of the standing wave then couples with and drives the amplitude of all internal physiological processes.[4]

The Control Interrupt Model posits that these spirit voices are the nonlinear artifacts of the hallucinogenic interrupt frequency overlapping into multisensory frame perception with a specific ADSR (attack, decay, sustain, release) envelope. By modulating standing vocal waves, the shaman can exactly match the periodic frequency of the hallucinogenic interrupt; by changing the shape of the lips, the speed of air through the glottis, and the speed of the tongue flicking towards the back of the throat, the shaman can replicate the slippery shape and feel of the hallucinogen's interrupt envelope. Resonance is a term applied to oscillators when the shape and frequency of one standing wave harmonizes with and drives the amplitude, or energy, of another standing wave. By using the physical techniques of sound shaping and resonance, the shaman can amplify the hallucinogenic interrupt of any psychedelic and, beyond that, drive standing wave coherence among multiple participants in a shamanic ritual. This process is intuitive if the shaman merely pays close attention to his or her internal physiology as the hallucinogen takes action.

In the nomenclature of chaos theory, when a chaotic system evolves towards a particular state over time, that state is called an attractor, or a strange attractor in fractal systems. According to PIT, nonlinear consciousness is multi-stable, which means it can have many strange attractors pulling it towards many different stable states; or it can become stuck in a superposition or chaotic phase transition between two or more stable attractors. In normal perception, the primary attractor is linear consciousness; when consciousness is dramatically perturbed it will always find a way to return to the linear state after enough time, and consciousness tends to return to the linear state even when momentarily destabilized. In nonlinear consciousness the attractor may be a manic state, a trance state, a disoriented state, a paranoid state, an enlightened state, and so on. As psychedelic consciousness becomes complex and bifurcates, it gradually moves towards one of many multi-stable attractors, eventually locking into a complex stabilized state based on periodic drivers in set and setting. Once a subject under the influence of psychedelics finds an attractor state and locks into it, it becomes difficult to break the stabilizing harmonic pattern to move towards another attractor. Navigating between strange attractors in the destabilized nonlinear state is the primary function of shamanic singing and ritual; without the ability to self-navigate to a specific attractor, the subject may become stuck in a negative attractor, like an anxiety spiral or paranoid feedback loop.

Control Interrupt and Spirit Spaces

Mixing the Control Interrupt Model with traditional shamanic metaphors, it is accurate to say that the spirit world of each hallucinogen is literally erupting or interrupting into normal consciousness by carving out a distinct wave space where spirits can sneak packets of information to the subject in between normal frames. In physical terms, spirit information erupts into consciousness along the attack and decay of each psychedelic interrupt, then attenuates salient recognition and imprints itself into memory according to the receding sustain and release. As the interrupt's interference pattern overlaps onto multisensory perception, spirit information will appear to overlap onto the fabric of reality; bending towards the subject from a nearby dimension; trickling or gurgling over an invisible spillway; flickering in a stroboscopic film reel; parting through folds in a lattice or screen; becoming visible underneath a silken veil; and so on.[6] The subjective view of the spirit world is that it is an "invisible landscape" suddenly made visible to human eyes, and the addition of the hallucinogenic driver allows the veil of perception to be drawn open like shutters. These are all allusions to the boundaries of perceptual space changing as the hallucinogenic interrupt gains power, entrains sensory processing networks, and generates complex interference patterns.

To clarify this process with a metaphor, in the realm of shamanism it may be helpful to think of serotonergic (5-HT) modulation as reality, and the frequency of the hallucinogen as the spirit world. If serotonergic reality is modulated in the beta range at 12-30 Hz, and the hallucinogenic interrupt of tryptamine Y is modulated to 24 Hz, then there will be a predictable 24 Hz frame flicker superimposed over normal perception when you ingest hallucinogen Y. The interrupt frequency of 24 Hz presumes a very fast pulsation, fast enough to produce film-like or fully animated cartoon hallucinations. The 24 Hz spirit interrupt then masks itself onto multisensory pathways and is perceived as an ontologically distinct spirit realm emerging as a phantom but embedded part of physical reality. The physical intensity and tactile sensuality of the hallucinogenic spirit overlay will depend on the speed, shape, and intensity of the molecule's ADSR interrupt; higher doses of hallucinogen typically means harder attack, longer sustain, elongated release, and more seamless merging between reality and hallucination.

Driving Interrupt Amplitude and ADSR Transitions

As a psychedelic chemical is ingested and metabolized, the frequency and ADSR envelope of the hallucinogenic interrupt will transition over time. This shift in modulatory interrupt can be described as a change in interrupt amplitude over duration of effect; higher amplitude of interrupt means stronger and more realized hallucinations. A shaman will instinctively modulate the tones of his or her chants and songs to match the interrupt frequency and envelope of the hallucinogen as it begins to take effect. This technique accurately describes the oscillating drones, throat singing, slurping, sucking, squelching, whooshing, whistling, guttural ululating, and other vocalizations associated with ayahuasca shamanism.[2,3] If a shaman can drive interrupt amplitude through constructive vocal interference he or she should also be able to dampen interrupt amplitude through destructive vocal interference.[5] This technique would manifest as the ability to snap a subject out of an intense psychedelic experience with a quick change in phase between vocal waves and hallucinogenic interrupt frequency to decrease and flatten interrupt amplitude.

Techniques of using resonance to drive and shape wave amplitude have been exploited by modern DJs and music producers to engineer hard-attack bass lines associated with acid house and trance music. In the psychedelic musical genre known as Goa Trance, bass lines rip through crowds of thousands of dancers with the resonant wave shape and amplitude of electric saw blades. The intensely amplified resonant pulse drivers of Goa Trance music are, in fact, the current bleeding-edge ritual technology of physical shamanism. Goa Trance originated from India; Goa Trance DJs and producers are revered like gurus or techno-shamen; and fans of Goa Trance travel to global music festivals the way other spiritual adherents make yearly pilgrimages. Goa Trance music is the psychedelic essence of resonant hallucinogenic tryptamine interrupt expressing itself through modern ritual entrainment technology. Using an electrically amplified sound system, a trance DJ can manipulate a tribe of thousands in the same way a traditional shaman manipulates a tribe of dozens (Fig. 25). It is shamanic folk technology now applied on an industrial scale.

Cellular Automata and Fractal Imprinting

It may be difficult to understand how a simple periodic interrupt or modulatory frame pulse can create such dramatic perceptual results, but the hallucinogenic interrupt should be thought of as a linear resonant driver which, over time, generates complex and salient wave interference patterns. This can also be described by a dynamical information processing system generating complexity over time based on a simple repetitive algorithm, such as a fractal or a cellular automata. Fractals or cellular automata are perhaps the best visual metaphors for the spontaneous recursive organization of psychedelic visual hallucinations, and there is a very fractal or cellular element to the psychedelic experience which evolves along the flickering pulsation of the hallucinogen's interrupt. The endless unfolding of the infinite psychedelic fractal continues until the hallucinogen is metabolized, at which point the hallucinogenic interrupt wears off, fades away, and consciousness unwinds from the recursive spiral and stabilizes back into linear information processing.

Biology is repetitive feedback patterns; consciousness is repetitive feedback patterns; shamanism is the interruption and re-modulation of those repetitive feedback patterns to produce spectacular experiential results. In a very real way, shamanism is the art of shaping the fractal integrity of the individual from the genetic level up through personal memory and tribal identity. The hallucinogenic interrupt allows the shaman to break the subject's habituated daily routines and place them into a self-referential programming loop that includes all layers of personal and transpersonal identity. The interlocking facets of biological-self and transpersonal-self are made explicit in the flickering spirit space, and by controlling the depth of immersion into this space the shaman can control how much of the subject's existing identity is exposed, manipulated, and transformed in the process.

The fractal rendering of sub- and meta- consciousness in the shamanic space allows psychedelics to have a profound long-term effect on identity-based neuroplasticity.[9] By applying a resonant multisensory driver that acts as a fractal generator for archetypal symbols in imagination, the psychedelic paradigms imprinted into memory appear to be more cosmic, transpersonal, holographic, and durable than sum of linear identity constructs imprinted over the average lifespan. To be clear, the nonlinear iterative nature of psychedelic hallucination exploits archetypal symbol rendering to bypass linear ego and imprint a recursive, holographic view of the transcendent self within a larger emergent cosmic reality. This idealized, holographic representation of the self may be considered more "real" than the actual self, perhaps even experienced as the essential self, genetic self, transpersonal self, or the eternal soul. The ability to produce and manipulate a representation of the idealized transpersonal self makes psychedelics viable in shamanic transformation, clinical therapy, and spiritual awakening.

The holographic image of idealized self does not emerge in a single moment or even in a single psychedelic session; the organization of a psychedelic meta-identity is a process that may take many hours of a single psychedelic session or possibly multiple psychedelic sessions to fully complete. However, once the self-activation of psychedelic metaprogramming and holographic imprinting takes hold, the subject may perceive their transformation to be an evolutionary expression of a hidden genetic instruction set, or a more perfect and cosmically mature version of the self emerging through spiritual cleansing and rebirth.[7] There is evidence that a single psychedelic session can enhance self-worth and have lasting beneficial impact on mood and outlook.[8] There is also evidence that psychedelics can be used to imprint pathological, antisocial, and delusional identity constructs.[9] Holistic identity expression is generally considered to be a positive spiritual technology, but it can also be used to manipulate anxiety and exacerbate pathological behavior. This duality is commonly expressed in the nomenclature of therapy vs. mind control, negative vs. positive neuroplasticity, or shamanism vs. sorcery and witchcraft.

Linear vs. Nonlinear Memory Imprinting

The limits of human memory present some challenges for accurately encoding or describing the information generated in psychedelic states. Waking memory encodes linear, semantic information; dreams encode associative eidetic information; psychedelics encode nonlinear fractal information. There are many factors which limit the ability to accurately remember or recall psychedelic information. The rush of information is too fast; the content of the experience is too ineffable; and the processes of dreaming and eidetic visual hallucination blocks the formation of new semantic memories. In order to remember a dream a subject must wake up and make some mental notes, then go back to sleep to finish the dream; but if the subject does not rouse to some level of lucidity the dream is almost always forgotten. The same can be said for psychedelic hallucination; if the subject is too overwhelmed to make mental notes, the content totally bypasses linear semantic memory. However, if psychedelic hallucination employs the same spontaneous organization of eidetic information used to encode associative long-term memory through dreaming, then psychedelic fractal information may also imprint directly into long-term memory at a subconscious level.

Shamanic Information Compression

The functional limitations of human memory and expression have been problematic for high-dose psychedelic research from the beginning. The best writing, artwork, and video emulating the psychedelic experience must be created after the fact, sometimes painstakingly so. The visual reconstruction of psychedelic memory is a labor intensive process; a single subjective psychedelic frame may take weeks or months to visually render, and will still be lacking in context and complexity from the original experience. This is even more frustrating when you consider that a one line fractal algorithm or cellular automata can generate enough novel artistic complexity to keep the average human fascinated for hours. Linear approaches to capturing the psychedelic aesthetic almost always pale in comparison to their simpler, nonlinear generative counterparts.

The one artistic medium which can be expressed immediately in psychedelic intoxication without disrupting the quality of the shamanic experience is music. A shaman can relate the tone and content of the psychedelic experience in real time by singing, vocalizing, or playing drums (Fig. 26); this is the traditional method for binding psychedelic memory into physical space. The act of singing, drumming, or dancing also drives feedback and amplifies the energy of the psychedelic experience, thus making music the primary medium of psychedelic information compression and transmission.

There is compelling evidence that spontaneous singing and vocalization are forms of nonlinear psychedelic information compression. Glossolalia, or speaking in tongues, is reported as a spiritual side effect of psilocybin. Glossolalia may be considered a form of nonlinear speech, or psychedelic information erupting spontaneously through psycho-verbal synesthesia. When the shaman wants to speak with the spirit voice, that voice comes out more like music or glossolalia than like words and grammar. When a subject on psychedelics listens to music, the music expands from auditory signal into full multisensory synesthesia; every layer of emotional resonance in the song is laid bare for the subject to intimately see and feel. Claiming that psychedelics make music sound better or allow you to "see the music" is easy; this appreciation has fueled global music festivals and DJ circuits for decades. Shamanic music does not need to store visual information because under the influence of psychedelics the music naturally expands into visual perception. A sacred song from a rainforest shaman may not induce a strong reaction in a sober subject, but under the influence of ayahuasca that same song may open a window into the shaman's spirit world. This phenomena goes beyond the level of mere music appreciation, it demonstrates a cross-cultural technology for real-time encoding and transmission of nonlinear psychedelic information.

By examining the wave properties of ayahuasca *icaros*, is it possible to construct an experiential rendering of the synesthetic hallucinogenic effects. A shaman may make gurgling or retching noises to amplify modulatory interruption of 5-HT receptors in the gut to drive purgation. A fast rustling or shushing noise, like a snake rattle or wind through tree branches, evokes alpha-range relaxation and mental fluidity, and may also create goose-bumps and a salient sense of supernatural mystery. A droning drum beat or chant drives theta-band trance and hypnagogic states. A whistling or high pitched melody drives beta and gamma coherence, creating sharp multisensory synesthesia of rising eidetic images. A guttural croaking or a resonant bass line amplifies the saturated attack and decay of stacking hallucinogenic frames.

A shaman may employ one or all of these techniques at various stages of ceremony, and may use them repetitively or cyclically, like a winding stem that moves through deeper and deeper layers of hallucinogenic immersion. The shamanic technique of lulling and evoking mystical hallucination can be compared to the frenetic qualities of modern trance music, where the goal is to entrain and sustain a high-energy visual state that unfolds and recourses for extended periods of time. Trance songs are built around arpeggiated looping melodies which grow in complexity over time, culminating in phase transitions, or breakdowns, where stable looping states are shattered into chaos. While trance dancing, these breakdowns are felt as euphoric, like shattering a barrier into a higher state of freedom and bliss, and when the chaos of the breakdown converges back towards a rhythm, it is an even more frenetic level of organized syncopated beats driven and held together by deep resonant bass pulses. The wave analysis of both modern trance music and traditional *icaros* indicates that these are not merely forms of artistic expression, but are also formal technologies for mediating and navigating various levels of stability in chaotic psychedelic hallucination.

Notes and References

1. See Chapter 06, "The Control Interrupt Model of Psychedelic Action".

2. Beyer, SV, "Singing to the Plants: A Guide to Mestizo Shamanism in the Upper Amazon". University of New Mexico Press (October 31, 2009).

3. Observations of shamanic rituals and vocalizations taken from first-hand and recorded accounts of shamanic ceremonies.

4. Subjective reports of psychedelic intoxication include references to internal physiological processes achieving a dramatic synchronized efficiency. It is unknown if psychedelics have a globally coherent effect over all physiological processes, but since there are 5-HT receptors distributed throughout the entire body it is certainly within the realm of possibility.

5. WikiPedia.org, "Interference (wave propagation)". Internet Reference, 2010.

6. Descriptions of entering into the spirit world or receiving information through a lattice, veil, or spiritual overlay taken from subjective reports.

7. Themes of spiritual cleansing and rebirth are common in shamanism and psychedelic mysticism. Modern interpretations of these themes include genetic self-activation or evolutionary manipulation of DNA via psychedelic catalyst. While these descriptions feel authentic, there is no evidence to indicate that psychedelics drive manipulation or programming at a genetic level.

8. Griffiths, R.R., "Psilocybin can occasion mystical-type experiences having substantial and sustained personal meaning and spiritual significance". Psychopharmacology (2006) 187:268–283.

9. Groups linked to the weaponized use of psychedelics include the Manson Family, the SLA, Aum Shinrikyo, the CIA, and the United States Department of Defense.

10. Yu Jiang, "Trajectory selection in multistable systems using periodic drivings". Volume 264, Issue 1, 13 December 1999, Pages 22-29.

11. Chizhevsky VN, Corbalan R, "Multistability in a driven nonlinear system controlled by weak subharmonic perturbations". phycon, vol. 2, pp.396-402, 2003, International Conference on Physics and Control.

12. Charing HG, "Communion with the Infinite: The visual music of the Shipibo people of the Amazon". SH, Winter 2005.

Chapter 16

Physical Shamanism and Shamanic Therapy

The practice of spiritual shamanism and healing has been covered in many texts, so here we will examine physical models of shamanic therapy only as they apply directly to Psychedelic Information Theory (PIT). According to PIT, hallucination is the spontaneous production of nonlinear information via destabilization of multisensory perception.[1] Similarly, shamanic therapy is the production of spontaneous cellular organization via destabilization of metabolic homeostasis. An M.D. may prescribe a specific therapy to treat a specific symptom or pathology; a shaman will look beyond the pathology and prescribe radical dieting and psychedelic drug therapy to fully reboot, re-tune, and recycle the patient's entire metabolic process. Shamanic therapy can be considered a nonlinear or holistic approach to diagnosis and healing.

Modern Shamanic Psychotherapy

In modern clinical therapy psychedelics are employed to improve psychological resilience in the face of stress or trauma, typically in the case of depression, PTSD, and anxiety. Psychedelics are thought to produce psychological resilience through the spontaneous creation of autobiographical insights and transpersonal spiritual epiphanies which compress existing memories into a new holistic identity. According to PIT, the generation of salient insights in psychedelic trance is the byproduct of nonlinear information creation and memory compression, just as dreaming is a form of associative information creation and compression.[2] Even a single low-dose psychedelic session can produce changes in identity and transpersonal awareness that last a lifetime.[3,4,5]

To apply simple psychedelic therapy, the shaman need do nothing more than provide the medicine and a warm quiet place for the subject to lie down. Psychological resilience is generated by allowing the subject to navigate anxieties, forgive and accept past behaviors, and sense a transpersonal unity and love flowing through all creation. This method works best in targeted therapy, and should only be applied in a controlled setting to reduce anxiety spirals and negative plasticity.

Shamanic Dieting, Purging, and Cleansing

Traditional shamanic therapy typically includes components of restrictive dieting, fasting, and purgation of bodily wastes and fluids.[6] The common wisdom is that dieting and purgation cleanses and purifies the body, restoring it to harmony and balance. A more cynical analysis concludes that radical dieting and fasting destabilizes the body's metabolic homeostasis and puts it into deprived states of heightened alertness and stress, states which can easily produce psychosis if prolonged for a day or more. Subjective reports of psychedelic use often include an initial period of stomach pain and intestinal discomfort preceding full psychedelic destabilization; this is because the psychedelic must interrupt 5-HT receptors in the gut before metabolic homeostasis can be fully uncoupled and re-tuned. Techniques of dieting and fasting speed and amplify the destabilizing effect of psychedelics on global metabolic homeostasis.

Metabolic Destabilization and Cellular Regeneration

The Control Interrupt Model posits that hallucinogens produce complex perceptual results through pharmacological interference of multisensory frame stability.[1] The same model applied to neural oscillators in a sensory network can be applied to cellular oscillators in an biological matrix. Many functions of metabolism and cellular signaling are modulated by 5-HT and dopamine; interrupting these signaling pathways will not only produce patterns of spontaneous neural organization, they will also produce patterns of spontaneous metabolic and cellular organization. For instance, 5-HT_{2A} receptors and serotonin have been shown to play a large role in mediating blood platelet aggregation.[10] Hallucinogens target 5-HT_{2A} receptors, and platelet aggregation is a fundamental immune mechanism. 5-HT_{2A}

activation has also been demonstrated to produce powerful anti-inflammatory effects in cardiovascular and soft tissues; and 5-HT_{2A} agonists like LSD may produce potent anti-inflammatory effects against TNF-a (tumor necrosis factor alpha), an autoimmune regulator which has been indicated in atherosclerosis, rheumatoid arthritis, psoriasis, type II diabetes, depression, schizophrenia, and Alzheimer's disease.[11]

Because the 5-HT_{2A} receptor is a G-coupled protein that promotes secondary transmission within the cell membrane, psychedelics that target the 5-HT_{2A} receptor can influence a wide variety of intracellular functions. The signaling pathways mediated by the 5-HT_{2A} receptor include the release of charged calcium ions (Ca^{2+}) and the activation of PKC and MAPK, protein kinases which transfer energy to proteins and enzymes that regulate cellular metabolism and proliferation. Coaxing cellular signaling pathways into patterns of spontaneous regeneration, anti-inflammatory, or autoimmune organization is at the root of all physical shamanic therapy. This model can be applied to neural inflammation, as in cluster headaches; emotional inflammation, as in PTSD; stress-related soft-tissue inflammation, as in fibromyalgia; or any systemic inflammation related to stress, chronic disease, and auto-immune disorders.

Subjects under the influence of psychedelics sometimes report feelings of being cleansed from the inside, like each cell is being polished and organized, and that waste and cellular debris are being expelled. This sensation has been compared to a radical auto-immune response, like computerized maintenance routine for de-fragmenting and optimizing cellular memory structures. Just as neural assemblies may be coaxed into becoming spontaneous nonlinear feedback generators, cellular signaling pathways may be coaxed into generating information via spontaneous energetic metabolic pathway testing, strengthening, and regeneration. Just as nonlinear hallucination may facilitate memory potentiation in the same way as dreaming, nonlinear metabolic organization may facilitate cellular regeneration or immunological response similar to states of fever or deep restorative sleep. The cellular regenerative power of psychedelics have only recently been demonstrated in scientific terms, but in shamanic models this restorative function is taken for granted.

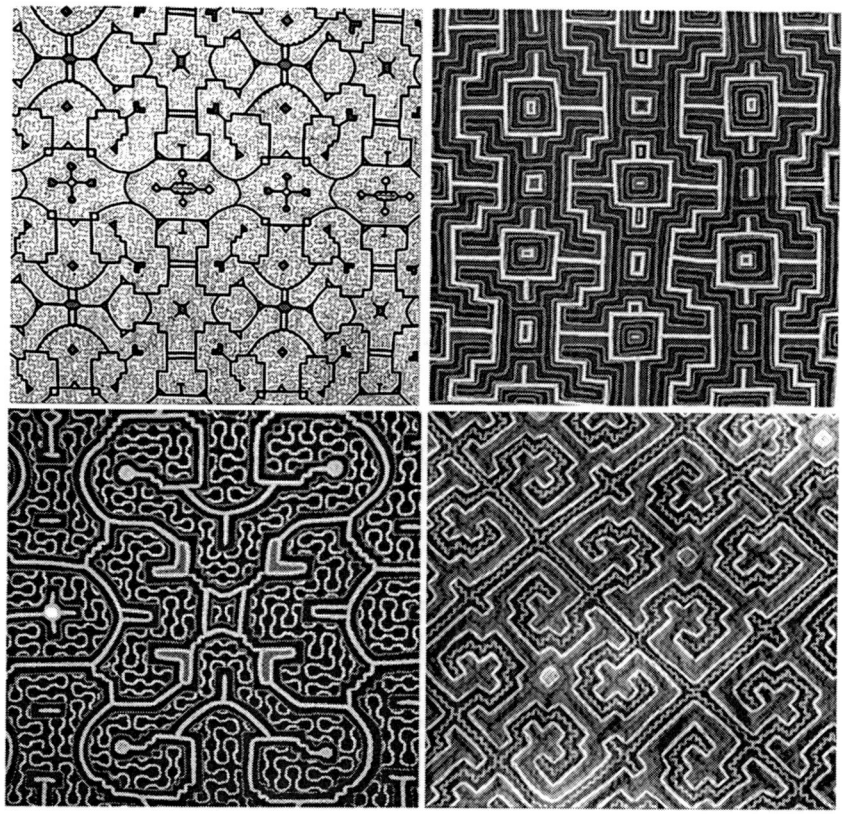

Figure 27. Patterns from Shipibo textiles are nonlinear artifacts of ayahuasca hallucination, and are also isomorphic of Chladni resonating interference patterns and Peano plane-filling fractal curves.

Physical Shamanism and Metabolic Entrainment

Physical shamanism employs wave-based entrainment techniques to coax spontaneous nonlinear organization in metabolic pathways and cellular signaling systems. Typical shamanic wave entrainment comes in the form of singing or music, but can also be applied through talk, touch, hypnotic motion, or other repetitive sensory feedback stimulation. Entraining a subject into a targeted state of consciousness is the science of hypnosis or trance. The psychedelic medicine allows the patient's homeostasis to become destabilized, and in this state the shaman becomes the circuit driver or entrainer, the oscillator with the most power to alter frequencies and amplify or dampen signal strength across the entire circuit. Acting as a hypnotic entrainer, the shaman can place the patient into dream-like trance and then synchronize his own perception to the patient's subtle internal body rhythms. The shaman uses the hallucinogenic interrupt as a control frequency for mediating contact with and manipulating the patient's metabolic processes. Once the control frequency connection has been established through mutual ingestion of the psychedelic medicine, the shaman then uses specialized entrainment waves to coax new metabolic interference patterns and signaling pathways throughout the patient's cellular matrix.

In Shipibo ayahuasca shamanism, the shaman takes the psychedelic medicine in order to visualize a flickering grid of patterns and symbols crawling across the surface of the patient. These ayahuasca patterns are embedded into Shipibo textiles (Fig. 27), ceramics, tattoos, and all forms of tribal artwork, and are considered to be visual representations of the *icaros* sung during shamanic ceremony. Each Shipibo pattern corresponds to a sacred psychedelic space where a specific type of information is manipulated and revealed, and by tuning the fluctuation of these patterns through the patient's biological systems, the shaman can sense blocked signaling pathways, restore atrophied pathways, and bring harmony and balance to the organism. Subjects under the influence of ayahuasca and shamanic singing often report the feeling of every cell in their body resonating in harmony with the healing songs of the *Maestro*.[7,8]

The ayahuasca shaman may employ hands-on techniques to massage the patient's energy patterns into a more harmonic shape, sometimes even sucking or blowing psychic energy through the patient, or perhaps performing a psychic surgery to remove a dark body, a block, or a curse.[9] Sometimes the shaman must dig very deep into muscle and organ tissue before the source of illness can be found; sometimes the patient's energy pathways are so blocked or degraded they are impossible to fix. The shaman may use high-pitched vocal tones to focus sound waves deep into the body, hoping to break apart blocked signal pathways via the power of resonant intonation. The shaman may use high pitched whining or whistling tones focused at one area of the body, or may use throat singing to invoke deep rumbling bass tones which make the patient's chest cavity resonate at same frequency as sound vibrations moving deep into the Earth.[7]

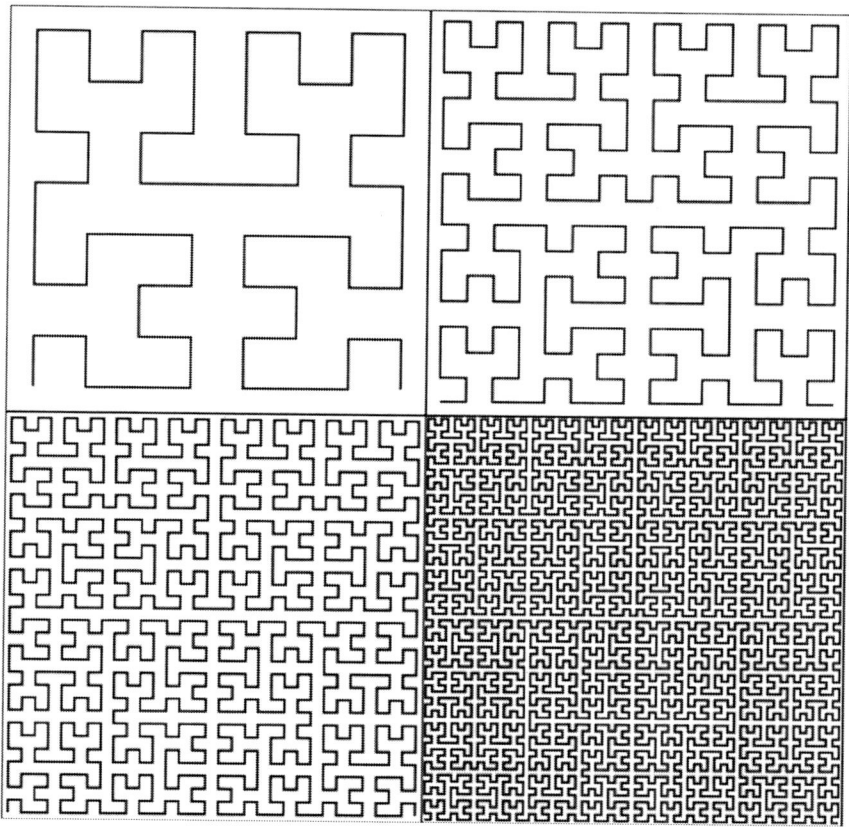

Figure 28. Hilbert curves are examples of recursively constructed L-shaped Peano curves, also called space-filling or plane-filling curves, which recede in granularity with each octave or iteration. From Wolfram Math, 2010.

The case can be made that Shipibo textile patterns and sacred songs are compressed artifacts of nonlinear hallucination. These patterns are isomorphic of Chladni resonating interference patterns (Fig. 31), as well as Peano space-filling fractal curves (Fig. 28), S- or L-shaped patterns which repeat in embedded granularity depending on the depth of system iteration.[12] Shipibo textile patterns correspond to specific resonating tones and states of consciousness, and *icaros* are cultural technologies for accessing specific states of highly organized nonlinear feedback complexity in both neural and cellular signaling pathways. By employing these techniques under the influence of psychedelics, the shaman can entrain the biological functions of the patient all the way down to the cellular level, perhaps even to the genetic level. Transitioning through these levels would depend on the granular complexity of the interference pattern, or depth of system iteration, created between the shamanic entrainment wave and the hallucinogenic interrupt.

Notes and References

1. See Chapter 06, "Control Interrupt Model of Psychedelic Action".

2. See Chapter 13, "Psychedelic Neuroplasticity".

3. Doblin, R, "Pahnke's 'Good Friday Experiment' A Long-Term Follow-Up And Methodological Critique". The Journal of Transpersonal Psychology, 1991, Vol. 23, No. 1.

4. Griffiths, R.R., "Psilocybin can occasion mystical-type experiences having substantial and sustained personal meaning and spiritual significance". Psychopharmacology (2006) 187:268–283.

5. Griffiths RR, Richards WA, et al., "Mystical-type experiences occasioned by psilocybin mediate the attribution of personal meaning and spiritual significance 14 months later". Journal of Psychopharmacology, Vol. 22, No. 6, 621-632 (2008).

6. Tindall R, "The Jaguar That Roams the Mind". Park Street Press, Vermont, 2008.

7. Charing HG, "Communion with the Infinite: The visual music of the Shipibo people of the Amazon". Eagle's Wing, Winter 2005.

8. Pantone, DJ, "The Shipibo Indians: Masters of Ayahuasca". Internet Reference, 2006.

9. Beyer, SV, "Singing to the Plants: A Guide to Mestizo Shamanism in the Upper Amazon". University of New Mexico Press (October 31, 2009).

10. Cerrito E, et al., "5HT2-receptors and serotonin release: Their role in human platelet aggregation". Life Sciences Volume 53, Issue 3, 1993, 209-215.

11. Yu B, et al., "Serotonin 5-HT2A Receptor Activation Suppresses Tumor Necrosis Factor-α-Induced Inflammation with Extraordinary Potency". JPET November 2008 vol. 327 no. 2 316-323.

12. Wolfram Math, "Peano Curves". Internet Reference, 2010.

Chapter 17

Hypnotic Entrainment and Induced Trance States

The fundamentals of hypnosis and induced trance states begin with the concepts of wave resonance and entrainment. Resonance is the quality of any oscillating system (waves in a neural network) to reach maximum amplitude (power) when stimulated with periodic drivers (pulses) at a specific pitch or rhythm (a resonant frequency). Oscillators can have many resonant frequencies which top out at maximum amplitudes. If we envision the brain as an oscillator for maintaining stable bands of consciousness, each band in the spectrum must therefore have its own corresponding resonant frequency, or frequencies, which can drive spontaneous phase transitions into that standing wave state. The process of using resonance to drive the frequency and amplitude of oscillators is called entrainment, and when the shaman induces a trance state he is applying resonant wave interference to entrain the frequency of the patient's neural oscillators.

Neural Oscillators

All states of consciousness are created by the act of neurons firing in a network. When a single neuron fires once it is not a big event, but when a neuron fires in a rapid sequence then it is signaling other neurons with a fine vibration of wave spikes; these neural spikes are the language of consciousness. When two or more neurons fire at the same frequency they are said to be synchronized, and when two areas of the brain are firing in synchrony there is said to be coherence between these areas, which means they are most likely engaged in a complex distributed processing task. When neurons are coupled together in a recurrent network, the rapid pulses sent back and forth between them are referred to as oscillations, and these oscillations take on the predictable mathematical properties of waves; a wave being any standing oscillation passing through a medium. These standing oscillations – literal waves of energy rippling through pathways in the cranial saltwater – are the field effect of consciousness flowing through the neural network. Smooth or harmonic propagation of these waves indicates high fidelity and stability in the field of consciousness; erratic propagation or interference in these waves indicates a chaotic, transitional, or destabilized field of consciousness.

EEG and Brainwaves

The wave-like oscillations of the brain can be measured via electroencephalography (EEG), a technique in which electrodes are placed on the skin and scalp to aggregate the voltage of energy waves produced along the outermost cortical layers of the brain. EEG machines produce graphs of brain activity over time, and each state of consciousness occupies its own distinct space along the brain wave spectrum (Fig. 29). The normal waking consciousness we perceive as active self is a beta state which begins around 12 Hz, or 12 cycles-per-second; this is the speed at which consciousness updates in a focused, active state. In highly focused or intense waking states these beta rhythms can be pushed up to around 38 Hz, which means the neural network would be cycling information at a rate of thirty-eight frames-per-second (FPS).

Below beta is the alpha state, in the 7-12 Hz range, which is associated with detached critical analysis and more relaxed physical intuition. Even more relaxed than alpha is the theta state between 4-7 Hz; this band makes up the transitional states between waking and sleeping, including meditative and lucid dream states. The waking mind finally shuts down at the delta range of 0.5 to 4 Hz, where the brain slows into the deep rhythms of regenerative sleep. The brain wave spectrum from 0.5 to 38 Hz is where we spend all of our days every day, with global brain cohesion rarely tipping over into the high gamma range of 40 Hz and beyond, bands associated with fast personal awareness and highly focused connective insight. But even higher than gamma is the hypergamma range, which is over 100 Hz; and above that is the mythical lambda state, over 200 Hz, where it is rumored that human consciousness tops out at total awareness of all things from the beginning of time to the end of history. On the other end, even lower than deep delta sleep, is the mythical epsilon state where brain waves drop below 0.5 Hz and a yogic state of suspended animation occurs.

When evaluating brainwaves, human consciousness appears to be like a musical instrument than can be tuned and tweaked along a predictable spectrum of possible tones and chords. The brain wave spectrum as detailed here is only the most basic information, but EEG and brain wave science is rich with detail on how the various states interact with one another. For instance, there is evidence that slow wave oscillators in the brainstem may act as the circadian drumbeat of all consciousness; that fast gamma waves are employed spontaneously to bind coherence between slower brain areas; that slow epsilon waves may drive amplitude in the hypergamma and lambda ranges; that the mu rhythm (8-12 Hz) controls and interprets contralateral motor activation; that there are specific brain organs and hormones responsible for attenuating specific pulse ranges and keeping the brain in synch; that beta states promote anxiety; that the brain constantly produces many simultaneous bands of activity at differing power ranges in any state of consciousness; and so on. Brainwaves are often fleeting, irregular, and disorganized; consciousness is distributed and constantly transitioning between multiple tasks and states of focus.

Hypnosis, Induced Trance States, and Entrainment

Most shamanic work is done in what is known as a trance state; a highly relaxed state of extremely narrowed focus. The traditional shamanic trance state is in the theta range, around 4-7 Hz, which is a meditative state in the boundary zone between sleeping and waking. Most shamanic drum circles drop naturally into the theta range, and this is the same range a hypnotherapist will drop a patient into when inducing a highly relaxed state. This range is also associated with daydreaming, memory recall, and guided visualization. The high end of the theta band is associated with internal focus, visualization, and sustained concentration; the lower end is associated with more transient states of daydream, spontaneous memory recall, and lucid dreaming. Somewhere in the lower end of this zone is the hypnagogic grey area between waking and sleeping where body-consciousness disappears and the user feels floating sensations and may have out-of-body experiences (OBEs).

One of the ways a shaman achieves a trance state is through hypnosis. A typical hypnotherapy routine will guide the patient slowly down through a relaxed alpha state and gently place them right on the borderline of the hypnagogic theta state. With the patient teetering on the edge of hypnagogia, the therapist can then either engage them casually in a minimally aware alpha state or tip them into an internal theta state where it is easier to imprint new suggestions onto existing memory structures. If the hypnotherapist wants to make a strong imprint, he will introduce a suggestion in a receptive alpha state, then drop the patient into a low theta state to process the suggestion, then bring them back up to alpha to reinforce the suggestion, and then finally send them back down to low theta or slow delta sleep for further deep associative imprinting. This basic hypnotic routine is meant to focus the patient into the disengaged trance where rational override is shut down and the brain is vulnerable to suggestive memory imprinting. Most modern hypnotherapy focuses on behavioral imprinting, but the hypnotherapist may also uncover lost memories, imprint new memories, suggest the patient is floating, or take the patient on a guided visualization through a dream world. While performing trance work the shaman will tell the patient to remain completely still; this is to minimize circuit perturbation and wave interference produced by voluntary motor rhythms.

Shamanic Entrainment Technology

Hypnotherapy contains many of the same elements of shamanism, but hypnotherapy does not work for everyone. In shamanic therapy the psychedelic agent is applied to destabilize top-down control and make the patient more susceptible to entrainment for longer periods of time.

If the patient is lying down with their eyes closed then psychedelics will produce a trance state fairly reliably on their own; the shaman does not need to do much more than measure an accurate dose and provide a safe place for quiet reflection. But aside from treating patients, the shaman also leads group bonding rituals, and these group rituals all utilize similar hypnotic entrainment technologies.

Typical shamanic entrainment technology may include drums, chants, music, strobe lights, chimes, audio pulses, and talk routines which guide the ritual participants into a shared trance. Native American peyote rituals use the beat of a medicine drum as the synchronous driver for the baseline trance, and then layer the rhythm with vocal drones to create resonant drivers which maximize brain wave amplitude and global coherence in the group circuit. Discussion of periodic resonant oscillators and entrainment is essentially a physics-based deconstruction of music's power to induce and lock targeted mind states, which is something we all instinctively understand from the experience of listening to music. However, when you look at this dynamic from a physical standpoint, when the mind is entranced by an entrainment technology such as music, the mind and the music merge from separate individual oscillators into a standing harmonic interference pattern with its own unique properties of coherence and stability.

In traditional Amazonian ayahuasca ceremonies, the shaman may be blessed with an *icaro*, or a sacred song which is delivered spontaneously into the brain by the spirits. When the shaman sings this sacred song, the ritual participants are quickly ushered into the sacred space along with the shaman. Using the entrainment dynamic it is reasonable to assume to that these *icaros* are feedback vocalizations tuned to the resonant frequency of the specific trance state occupied by the shaman. The shaman hears the resonant frequencies in his head as hallucinogenic artifacts of the phase transitions happening within his neural oscillators, and when he vocalizes these noises they come out as pitched micro-tones, often layered with vibratos coming from the nose and throat. By layering resonant multi-tones into the sacred song, the shaman increases the amplitude and entrainment power of his neural and vocal oscillators. If the shaman and the ritual participants all sing the same tones together, their oscillators all merge into a constructive interference pattern and drive each other into a higher amplitude of shared energy. This is the physics of neural entrainment and linking group mind.

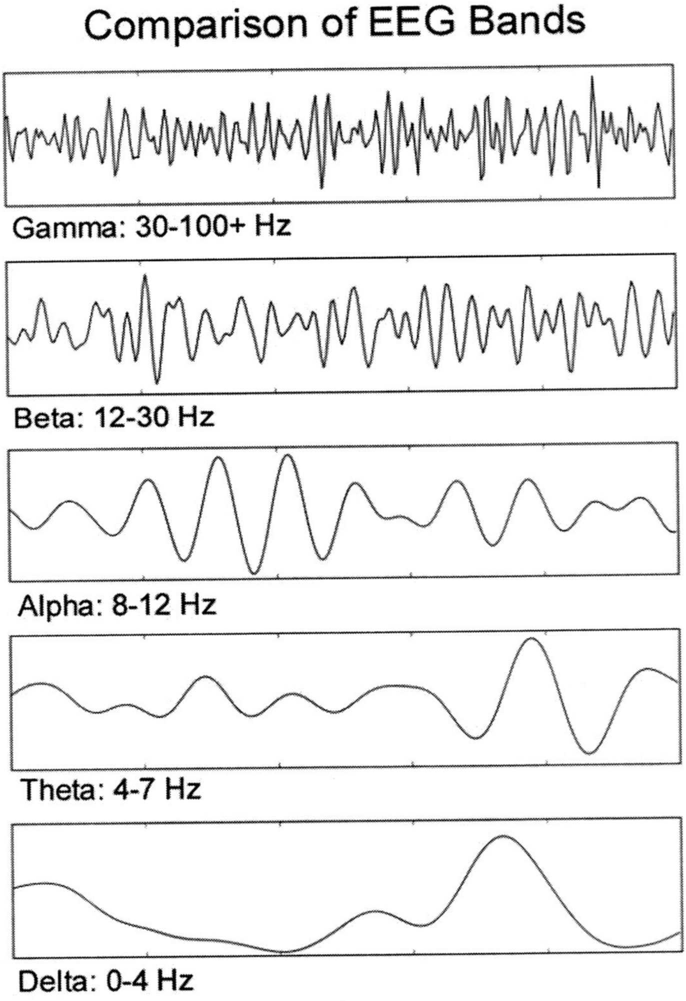

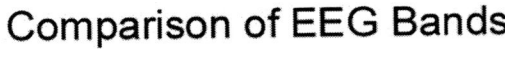

Figure 29. EEG bands over one second of activity. From WikiPedia.

Chapter 18

Psychic Bonding and Psi

Psychic bonding is a physical, neurological adaptation that occurs when two subjects spend time together sharing thoughts, feelings, and personal space. Psychic bonding is a survival trait that all animals and possibly all plants share. Psychic bonds can create personal vulnerabilities, so the average subject will have a built-in resistance to psychic bonding unless there is an explicit survival need and a certain level of trust established between subjects. Resistance to psychic bonding naturally breaks down over prolonged exposure between subjects living in the same confines as trust becomes routine and implied. In order to form a psychic bond, subjects must spend a period of at least a few hours together; a period of two to three days is optimal. Subjects should be together throughout all daily activities: waking, sleeping, eating, working, relaxing, etc. Sharing the schedules and routines of daily life is essential to synching the circadian rhythms and cross-expectations of each subject.

Psychic Bonding and Circadian Rhythms

Circadian rhythms are the master clock which controls all the state changes an organism undergoes in a 24-hour period. We wake up, get active, get hungry, get relaxed, get sleepy, go to sleep, and dream on a predictable cycle that mirrors the rotation of our planet, our moon, and our own internal biology. Subjects who are synched to the same circadian rhythms are locally bound to the same hourly oscillator, which means they share the same time-zone and daily living schedules. People who are called to perform daily routines at certain hours – like the prayer times of Islam, the coffee and lunch breaks of Western corporatism, or the hourly news cycles of modern media culture – have particularly high levels of local circadian binding. Usually circadian rhythms must be synched before psychic bonding between subjects can begin, though there is anecdotal evidence that psychic bonding can take place over telepresence if virtual contact is maintained for extended periods of time.

Psychic bonding usually takes place within a household; the household can be a metaphor for any group living situation, it can be an actual house, a business or partnership, or it can be a loose tribal structure like a band, team, squad, or similar nomadic crew. When living within close confinement, subjects are forced to work together, compromise, and share rigidly induced schedules for eating, relaxing, and sleeping. As subjects coexist they begin to build internalized constructs of each other which dictate how they behave and interact; these are cross-expectations fed by mirror neurons analyzing cooperative behaviors. The close familiarity between subjects drives a neural wiring process which embeds the patterns of each bonding partner into the other's mind, a process called mutual plasticity. Routine familiarity between subjects drives mutual plasticity.

Stress- and Pheromone-Induced Neuroplasticity

Smell is the most evocative of human senses because it is wired tightly into reward and fear responses, and of all the things that entice and repulse us about other people smell is arguably the strongest. When subjects are living in close proximity they produce hormones, pheromones, and they sweat, and when those pheromones are inhaled they produce instinctual emotional and neural responses. There is a very complex relationship between hormones, pheromones, behavior, mating, and bonding that permeates the entire plant and animal kingdom; it is a subject that transcends molecular biochemistry and approaches organic information field theory. Attempting to break down the non-verbal power of pheromones to induce bonding and neural growth can lead to many interesting digressions, but what is most germane to our discussion is that when humans are under stress they produce hormones and they sweat, and that hormone-laced perspiration induces powerful empathetic responses in other humans. The feedback of pheromonal response between subjects over a period of a few circadian cycles will automatically drive the bonding process even if subjects are naturally resistant. The introduction of stress into the group household will increase hormonal response and thus make the bonding process more urgent and more powerful.

Bonding can be slow and relaxed, like the way a family builds familiarity over time; or it can be fast and forced like the way cults, fraternities, and militias haze subjects into coherence in a matter of days or weeks. Bonding can also be artificially induced through drugs, group mind rituals, or through the stress of surviving combat or a natural disaster with a small group of people. Bonding pairs are most likely mates, partners, roommates, or people who live and travel together in small tribe-like groups. Hostages can also bond with their captors in what is famously known as Stockholm syndrome,[1] which is an example of stress creating a situation where the brain is ripe for entrainment and imprinting.

A romantic version of group mind leading to psychic bonding might happen spontaneously on date when two potential mates sit and talk quietly for long periods of time, sharing vulnerable aspects of themselves over dinner, drinks, and conversation. If the couple is good fit, they will slowly synch into harmony with each other over the course of an evening until they wind up talking all night, feeling like they've never met anyone who understands them so deeply and intuitively. This is pheromones, proximity, and self-reinforcing neural feedback embedding instinctual rhythms in the rapport between two subjects; or neural cross-expectations. The overlap of hormonal response, brain wave coupling, and proximity between subjects will, over time, build strong synaptic connections which bind these individuals together.

Informational Capacities of Bound Partners

While the telepathic capacity of bound subjects is limited, a bound partner can still tell, for instance, what a partner is thinking just by looking at their face. The telepathy is generally not literal and symbolic, it is intuitive and empathetic. Bound partners will share intuitive rhythms of speaking and interacting – sharing phrases, inside jokes, and specialized facial expressions – and will spontaneously fall into these rhythms whenever they are together, even if they have been separated for long periods of time. There is constant anecdotal evidence that bound partners often spontaneously think of each other at the same moment, causing one to call or seek out the other just as the other thinks of doing the same; or that pets intuitively know when their owners are on the way home.[2] More intriguingly there is evidence indicating that bound partners can non-locally sense when the other is surprised, startled, or in danger.[3,4,5] Bonded pairs being synched on an intuitive level may not be literal telepathy, but this can definitely be classified as psi which has obvious survival advantages.

The key capacity of bonded pairs is that they can think and move fluidly as a pack and work instinctively with each other on an intuitive and non-verbal level. The demonstrable capacity for organisms to bond into collective groups emerges at the bacteria level and becomes most obvious at the insect or hive level. Through the mechanistic means of pheromones and receptors, insects can coalesce into a hive mind capable of many coordinated tasks; this is non-verbal cooperation based solely on encoded rules of instinctive behavior. Fish form schools, birds form flocks, mammals form packs, humans form tribes and towns and cities. Humans can also form psychic bonds with domesticated animals such as cats and dogs and horses, cross-encoding verbal and non-verbal communication for simplification of everyday needs and routines. There is also anecdotal evidence of people bonding with plants. The hormonal process for psychic bonding is genetically encoded and instinctual in cases of extended close proximity, intimacy, and stress; these are the exact variables needed for breaking or domesticating wild animals; the same variables needed for brainwashing; the same variables needed for cult indoctrination and deprogramming. The psychic bonding process is an instinctual evolutionary capability which can be exploited for positive or negative purposes, and the quality of information passed through psychic bonds can be described as automatic, self-stabilizing, non-verbal, advantageous, and intuitive.

Notes and References

1. WikiPedia.org, "Stockholm Syndrome". Internet Reference, 2010.

2. Sheldrake R, "A New Science of Life: The Hypothesis of Morphic Resonance". Park Street Press, Vermont. 1995.

3. Luke D, "Psi-verts and Psychic Piracy: The Future of Parapsychology". Reality Sandwich, Internet Reference, 7-6-09.

4. Richards TL, Kozak L, Johnson C, Standish LJ, "Replicable functional magnetic resonance imaging evidence of correlated brain signals between physically isolated subjects". Journal of Alternative and Complementary Medicine, 11, 955-963.

5. Kittenis M., Caryl PG, Stevens P, "Distant psychophysiological interaction effects between related and unrelated participants". Association 47th Annual Convention: Proceedings of Presented Papers, Vienna (67-76), 2004.

Chapter 19

Group Mind and Fluid Tribal Dynamics

The physical theory of group mind begins with some basic assumptions about oscillators and wave mechanics. If the mind is a resonant oscillator for processing information, and two oscillating minds can be synchronized through harmonic or resonant wave interference, then two minds entrained in a synchronized state should be able to pass information from one mind to the other. This theory sounds like potential telepathy, but the reality is more subtle and complex. The information that can be shared between oscillators is non-verbal and non symbolic; it exists in the realm of frequencies, wavelengths, and amplitudes. The most common information passed between entrained oscillators is synchrony testing and error correction, self-correcting mechanisms which maintain oscillator stability. Intuitive synchrony testing and error correction between two or more minds coupled in the same circuit is subjectively perceived as nonverbal communication, group mind, intuition, telepathy, or psi.

Examples of synchrony testing and error correction exist in all forms of communication. When information is flowing smoothly between oscillators, the data transfer has high speed and synchrony; when information transfer from one oscillator fluctuates and becomes ambiguous, the other instantly corrects to resolve the instability and regain synchrony. If automatic synchrony testing and error correction did not exist, any fluctuation in signal fidelity across the circuit would make the oscillator decouple. Synchrony testing and error correction can happen in a verbal conversation, a digital packet transfer, a cellular coding system, the harmonic chiming of bells, and so on. Synchrony testing and error correction allows entrained oscillators to retain stability through mutual feedback control, conserving or amplifying energy by phase locking into stable harmonic configurations. Individuals bound in a group activity use intuitive synchrony testing and error correction to maintain harmony through behavioral coordination and unitary cohesion.

Group Trance and Entrainment Technology

A practicing shaman must be a master of at least one ritual entrainment technology, and must be a master of putting himself and others into a targeted trance state; this is the bare minimum, the rest happens naturally. Some shaman simply provide total quiet and let the medicine do the work; some shamen put on elaborate shows which include singing, chanting, and live musical performance. The jam band phenomena started by adapting the dynamics of medicine drum circles to 1960s psychedelic party culture; hence the Grateful Dead and the growth of the Rainbow Family. In the 1990s the shamanic entrainment ritual was reduced to something as mundane as playing records on a loud stereo system with heavy bass, and this mundane task blossomed into the celebrity DJ profession which fuels modern global party culture. Any live performer can tell you that the feedback circuit between musician and audience fuels the energy of the performance, culminating in the moments when the performer and audience all sing the same chorus or move to the same beat in unison. It is the same with churches; it is the same with sporting events; it is the same with the military. When the audience participates in the performance, either dancing or clapping or singing in unison, it drives the amplitude of the entire circuit. This is spirituality, religion, and group transcendence reduced to wave mechanics.

There are two steps to entraining group mind. You must first demand focus of group attention, and then you must masterfully apply the entrainment technology; these rules are immutable and are the same for the hypnotherapist, the shaman, the musician, the salesman, the politician, the TV programmer, and so on. Demanding the attention of a large group of people is perhaps the hardest part, but the ritual entrainment technology can arguably be purchased at retail. In a club setting the focus of attention is commanded by the DJ, who applies prefabricated entrainment rhythms (dance grooves) to the crowd. When the crowd responds favorably to a specific groove by dancing with exuberance, the DJ rewards them by finding more grooves that fall into the same tempo, and then uses dynamic filters to isolate and boost the resonant frequencies of the walls in the room, pushing the music over the top with tremors that literally rattle the earth. When the DJ establishes a strong feedback control circuit with the crowd, there is phase transition where the crowd ceases to be individuals and they cohere into a single fluid unit. At this point the crowd becomes synchronized in audio-motor synesthesia with the music, almost like puppets (Fig. 25). The physical dynamics of a group of people engaged in trance dancing defies formal social descriptions and is best described as a coherent wave interference pattern.

Group Mind and Behavioral Phase Transitions

This spontaneous movement of a group of individuals into a coherent organism can be described in terms of phase transition from solid state to a liquid state of group dynamic. In the solid state there is ego, language, etiquette, social hierarchy, and rules of one-on-one engagement that keep individual identity separated and solid; in the liquid state individuals drop social pretenses and merge seamlessly into the flock, navigating instinctively via environmental cues and mutual feedback. When a group of individuals moves from a solid to a liquid state, there is a sense of transcendence that is subjectively perceived as joyful, cathartic, and spiritual. Subjects in a liquid group state feel unity, love, and purpose as the energy of the crowd flows through them like a transistor in an electrical circuit.

A similar example of social dynamics passing from solid to liquid state occurs in flocks of birds. On the ground birds assume pecking orders which create the dynamic for mating and nesting, in the air they become a fluid unit that navigates as a seamless whole. This social phase state transition is observable, repeatable, and may be measured generally in terms of global power across alpha bands of the entire group. In the ego-driven beta state the solid norms of society and hierarchy apply, but in the relaxed alpha state behaviors become more fluid and intuitive. In the beta state the individual is concerned only with fulfilling their own rational agenda; in the alpha state the individual moves seamlessly with the flow. When the tribe adopts a fluid social state it becomes a temporary autonomous zone for interpersonal experimentation, identity play, and other ego-blurring experiences that reinforce intimacy and group loyalty.

Informational Capacity of Group Mind

Shamanic mythology tells us that tribe members synchronized to group mind enter a telepathic dream-space where they can all share thoughts and visions. The sensation of bonding and becoming one with the group is real, but the level of telepathic ability achieved in group states is debatable. In a group trance the rational ego is detached and non-verbal intuition is fully engaged; empathy bonding is high and the hallucinogenic medicine turns group intuition into concrete visions. This enhanced non-verbal intuition can be called telepathy, psi, or a shared dream-space, but it would be wrong to assume that each member of the tribe is automatically sharing the same thoughts or visions just because they are all synchronized to the same hallucinogenic control wave or entrainment frequency.

The informational capacities of group mind are limited in a number of ways. Mutual feedback synchrony between peers coupled in group mind is nonverbal, local, and time dependent. At a distance peer and group coupling becomes weaker, and this coupling grows weaker the longer peers are separated by distance. Many traditional shamanic ceremonies recur weekly, or perhaps monthly with the phases of the moon. Shamanic ceremonies often employ the ritual of the medicine circle, a literal circuit of individuals bound in the ceremony for the duration of the ceremony. Breaking the circle in the middle of the ceremony is strongly discouraged, because energy shared and amplified in the circle can escape into the ether instead of staying within the group. Creating the sacred circuit on a recurring basis extends the power of non-local peer coupling over the periods between ceremonies, allowing for extended synchrony at a distance as long as the circuit binds locally or meets to synchronize at regular intervals. Recurring group circuits, such as shamanic ceremonies, church attendance, weekly business meetings, social clubs, and so on, reinforce instinctive behavioral cohesion and cross-expectations between group members.

Group mind can accurately be described as a form of distributed cognition, where the units of a group are coherently bound in a larger integrated system or process. From a distributed standpoint group mind is not literal telepathy, it is instead a form of cooperative thought emerging simultaneously as part of the coherent group process. Distributed functioning in the insect kingdom is commonplace; in the animal kingdom it takes the form of group movements like flocking, herding, and schooling, but sometimes emerges in more complex actions like hunting and stalking. The information shared in distributed tasking is limited to intuitive coherence of motor behavior to fulfill specific tasks and group functions. Behavioral cooperation and functional stability in group mind states is mediated through intuitive, nonverbal synchrony testing and error correction between coupled peers. In team sports and military operation, this highly intuitive group state is sometimes called being in "the zone."

Chapter 20

Shamanic Sorcery

Shamanic sorcery is the craft of manipulating the fabric of psychedelic space for personal gain or vendetta. Powers ascribed to shamanic sorcery include clairvoyance, spirit channeling, shape shifting, astral travel, remote viewing, curses, dream projection, magical darts, telepathy, mind control, necromancy, and so on. The shamanic ontology, or psychedelic spirit space, can be cynically viewed as a shared non-physical, non-temporal delusion accessible to any shaman as long as they accept the rules of the central ontology. In this way the shared shamanic ontology becomes fluid through space and time, and is magically manipulated and reinforced through ritual use of psychedelic drugs. In a setting where the shamanic ontology is readily accepted and reinforced, the shaman has great power; in reductive scientific settings that refute the shamanic ontology, the shaman appears to have an overactive guru complex and delusions of grandeur.

While PIT may appear to discount the claims of shamanic sorcery and spirit channeling, very few scientific studies have been done to either verify or refute the efficacy of psychedelic sorcery. A close reading of the literature on psychedelic discovery by the West reveals that scientists, therapists, and academics have rushed to exploit the power of native visionary ritual without properly considering the cross-cultural psychic backlash.[1,2,3,6] If the shamanic space is purely delusional then modern advocates have nothing to fear by exploiting traditional psychedelic ritual; but if the shamanic space is a transpersonal information field then it should also be considered a battlefield for waging information warfare. Modern advocates cannot embrace the entheogenic side of psychedelic spiritual communion while simultaneously ignoring the darker aspects of a truly transpersonal ontology. Like the internet, which allows peers to couple in unique ways, a shared shamanic network for sending and receiving information is also a vector for potential treachery and attack.

Sorcery and Nonlinear Influence

From a reductive standpoint, the shaman's magical influence is limited only to his tribe members, local neighbors, or those within his personal network; influence within this sphere is easy to account for in purely physical terms. From a metaphysical standpoint, the shaman is also said to be bound non-locally to all spirits and shamen in the psychedelic space regardless of physical or temporal location. The shaman is also said to be able to enter people's dreams, making the destabilized world of fleeting nocturnal visions like a global river for the shaman to navigate. These transpersonal claims are harder to account for in physical terms, and recent theory has attempted to tie the shamanic space to a non-local Akashic or morphogenetic field where non-physical spiritual or biological information is stored and transmitted.[4,5] A shared morphogenetic field should infer evolutionary advantage, but it also implies non-local vulnerability. Attack sorcery often requires a clipping of hair, a fingernail, a personal item, or a totem of the attack target. From a morphological perspective the sorcerer uses the genetic traces of these items as a resonating antenna to attack the target directly through the morphic field.

Under the influence of psychedelics, the shaman can hear the chattering of nonverbal information coming from the jungle, the city, the plants, the animals, and can intuitively sense the natural rhythms and cycles receding into the past and future. The shaman can blow a curse into the passing wind, or at a passing animal, and send magic darts on convoluted pathways towards enemies. From a nonlinear standpoint sorcery does not have to make rational sense. The placebo effect is a positive example of a nonlinear result that does not make rational sense; the same can be said for a curse that causes an enemy to suddenly fall ill. These results only make sense if you analyze them from a longitudinal perspective and follow the small periodic permutations of system variables as they produce disproportionately complex results through time; recovery in the case of placebo, or sickness and death in the case of a curse.

According to the fundamentals of Psychedelic Information Theory, the influence of shamanic sorcery can be presumed to be nonlinear, which means small periodic perturbations of system variables within a larger information system can produce disproportionately complex and chaotic results in any other part of the system. In the nonlinear psychedelic space the shaman is a chaos magician, or the butterfly that flaps his wings in China and creates a hurricane across the ocean. The nonlinear aspect of psychedelic sorcery makes it both a very subtle art form and something that escapes reductive scientific observation, but also makes it very prone to failure and lack of proper control. The weather is famously nonlinear, and one of the jobs of the shaman is reading and controlling the weather; this not a coincidence. PIT assumes that the study and mastery of nonlinear systems and emergent longitudinal complexity is a fundamental part of all psychedelic shamanism and sorcery.

Synchronicity Magic and Probability Collapse

Subjects in a destabilized nonlinear state often report enhanced sensations of non-random coincidence, or synchronicity, that appear to defy all rationality. Accounts of hidden forces acting in concert to send messages through non-random coincidence are common in psychosis, paranoia, schizophrenia, mania, bipolar disorder, and psychedelic intoxication. On psychedelics this state is dose dependent and increases in complexity with larger doses, until it appears the entire fabric of reality, down the subatomic level, is speaking directly to the subject with a singular narrative message. While in this "synchronicity hole," nothing in the universe seems random and all coincidence is laden with profound subtext that makes sense only to the subject. From a clinical standpoint, the synchronicity hole represents a state of delusional megalomania, yet this is exactly the kind of logic we should expect from a nonlinear analysis of reality. Linear analysis may perceive the leaves on a tree as a random distribution; a nonlinear analysis will see a singular non-random function underlying the genesis of complex form.

Subjective accounts of the synchronicity hole describe an immediate precognitive insight where probability appears to collapse and the subject intuitively knows exactly what is going to happen next. Another common description is that psychedelics open the mind to unlimited potential pathways into the future, and those potentials expand and collapse through time in direct response to the behaviors and will of the shaman. A shaman in this space is said to be able to look forward in time into many probable futures, and can choose any future simply by stepping into the vision and following the pathway that leads him there. By applying synchronicity magic and selecting non-random pathways into the future, the shaman expands and collapses probability and subtly alters the fabric of reality by choosing a new destiny. This process can be described in terms of deterministic chaos driving a superposition in subjective identity, leading to radical identity potentiation, behavioral change, and self-actualization through deterministic neuroplasticity.

Sorcery and Negative Information

According to PIT, shamanism is the craft of generating positive or stabilizing information within a larger matrix; sorcery is the craft of generating negative or destabilizing information within a larger information matrix. Negative information is any information which seeks to subvert or destroy parts or all of the larger information matrix. Examples of negative information at the biological scale include viruses, parasites, toxins, and cancers; at the personal scale negative information may include doubt, fear, stress, depression, abuse, neglect, trauma, and delusion; at the tribal level negative information may include dishonesty, distrust, withholding, disinformation, and warfare. When negative information is amplified with positive feedback, it can grow to destroy the entire system. Negative information can be countered with negative feedback, or dampened by positive information which seeks to bring stability back to the matrix. While a shaman uses psychedelics as a medicine or sacrament to heal and maintain tribal stability, the sorcerer uses psychedelics as a weapon to gain power over peers and attack enemies.

If shamanic sorcery is a kind of nonlinear chaos magic, it should also be considered to be somewhat unpredictable, uncontrollable, prone to high rates of failure, and potentially dangerous. Moreover, it is right to be suspicious of people interested in sorcery, which can be formally defined as negative information warfare waged for personal gain. Common wisdom dictates that when studying psychedelic shamanism one should learn under a *Maestro*, or master, who offers spiritual protection against black magic and sorcery.[3] While it is easy to dismiss these claims as superstition, the ambiguities and temptations of psychedelic sorcery have not been adequately addressed in the context of modern entheogenic ritual and clinical psychedelic therapy. Anyone experimenting in the field of psychedelic shamanism should be careful to avoid the dangers and temptations of sorcery.

Notes and References

1. Letcher A, "Shroom: A Cultural History of the Magic Mushroom". Faber, Great Britain, 2006.

2. Tindall R, "The Jaguar That Roams the Mind". Park Street Press, Vermont, 2008.

3. Beyer, SV, "Singing to the Plants: A Guide to Mestizo Shamanism in the Upper Amazon". University of New Mexico Press (October 31, 2009)

4. Oroc J, "Tryptamine Palace". Park Street Press, Vermont. 2009.

5. Sheldrake R, "A New Science of Life: The Hypothesis of Morphic Resonance". Park Street Press, Vermont. 1995.

6. Russell D, "Drug War: Covert Money, Power & Policy". Dan Russell, 1999-2000.

Chapter 21

Spirits and Spiritual Communion

Spirit contact is a central part of many psychedelic practices. While the autonomy of spirit entities is a subject for endless metaphysical debate, the reports of seeing spirits under the influence of psychedelics are common enough to make some generalizations. First, psychedelic entities are anthropomorphic interfaces through which psychedelic information is generated or transmitted. Second, formal spirit types represent idealized versions of specific information matrices: cellular, insect, plant, animal, ancestral, mythic, alien, pagan, machine, cosmic, and so on, and each type of spirit reveals different insights into the ordered nature of life and the universe. Third, psychedelic spirits are tricksters; they often speak in riddles, communicate in visual rebus and pantomime, and typically never give a straight answer to inquiries. From an information standpoint it does not matter if the spirits are real or delusion, the information they generate is real and can be analyzed from a formal perspective.

Habits and Customs of the Spirits

A study of the literature on shamanism and helper spirits tells us many things about their behaviors and habits. First, spirits do not generally like light; they will occasionally appear in the daytime, but they prefer to appear in dim light, at night, in an area illuminated only by candle or firelight. Second, spirits usually come only when you call them, only after you have called them, in the long moments of silence following the request for them to appear. Third, spirits do not like loud noises; keeping the entire local area perfectly quiet is the only way to ensure they will feel safe to appear. Fourth, spirits do not like foul smells, they are drawn to the perfumed scents of tobacco smoke and various types of incense, and are repulsed by the smell of meat-eating humans, alcohol drinking humans, and menstruating women; foul smells may actually summon harmful spirits or demons. Finally, some spirits require that the shaman grovel, chant, sing, and produce offerings before they appear; this is not always required but is common enough to be considered typical. To call in the spirits the shaman must respect all these customs while taking large amounts of the psychedelic medicine. The spirits will only come if the shaman calls them at the proper time and place, after he has dieted and purged, taken the medicine, and then burned enough tobacco or incense to make the scent of the area meet stringent requirements. [1]

The ritual for calling the spirits includes many telling details. Fasting and a low-sugar, low-protein diet implies physiological tuning for destabilizing metabolic homeostasis. The doses of hallucinogen taken in spirit communion are high, typically twelve or thirteen pairs of psilocybin mushrooms for traditional Central American ceremonies. Ritual intonation of calling in the spirits, or requesting for them to appear in chant or song, sets the initial conditions for the hallucinogenic experience which follows. Stillness, low light, and silence offers the best conditions for acetylcholine modulation of the midbrain associated with sleep onset, which is known to produce dream-like imagery. Tobacco excites cholinergic modulation of the midbrain. Incense excites olfactory reward centers in the midbrain; foul smells excite olfactory anxiety centers and naturally produce visions that are more demonic than angelic. Psychedelics interfere with smooth muscle contractions related to digestion and uterine cramping, making hallucinogen use potentially uncomfortable for menstruating women, and potentially dangerous for pregnant women. The final element in the ritual is having faith that the spirits will appear, which reinforces the intonation and expectation that they will. And, surprisingly enough, if you follow the ritual exactly and have faith, the spirits will appear.

Interfacing with Spirit Information

If the shaman follows ritual protocol, ingests the psychedelic medicine, and manages to summon the spirits, he should not waste time bothering them with mundane questions. The spirits will typically answer only one question or perform only one task, and that task should be considered urgent and worthy of their participation or they will promptly dismiss the shaman and will not appear again for the rest of the session, perhaps not again for many weeks or months. Spiritual dismissal is reported often enough to be considered typical, so the formal spiritual quality of being offended by mundane inquiries should be noted when attempting to access spirit intelligence. By all accounts, forging reliable relationships with specific spirit entities takes time and requires a fair amount of dedication to learning their habits and ways. The information in the spirit matrix should not be considered a database you simply plug into and access like the internet, but more like a network of individuals whose trust you must gain and keep over a lifetime in order to share their wisdom. Traditional shamen report that one of the worst things that can happen is for the spirits to stop appearing because the shaman has lost his power or offended them in some way. Staying on good working terms with the spirits is a core theme of shamanism and retaining shamanic power.

Gnosis, the All One, and Nonlinear Communion

Subjective accounts of psychedelic transcendence often include reports of a cosmic connection to a single unified force, a force which sometimes speaks to or through the subject. This force does not appear physically or anthropomorphically, but instead appears to be imbued in the fabric of all things. Typically the subject is meditating, is lying still, is engaged in breathing exercises, or has a similarly detached focus when the voice begins to speak. When this force speaks it is through a layered nattering and murmuring arising from seemingly random and unrelated background noises. In a destabilized state, these random background noises synchronize into a coherent pattern of linear, directed communication from one fundamental source. When the fundamental source energy senses the subject's heightened awareness, it begins to coalesce and speak through his or her mind. This voice typically introduces itself in the subject's language with the slowly repeating phrase, "I am the All One, all that is, was, and will ever be."[2]

The All One is subjectively perceived as the mind, consciousness, will, and intent of the physical universe. There is often a sense of reverence, love, acceptance, and unity infused with the contact. Formal accounts of communion with the All One date back to the origins of Hermeticism and Gnosticism, and depict a pantheistic, teleological view of the universe as the sacred physical body of an ever-evolving omniscient God. Formal accounts of the All One clearly depict the scale of timeless omnipresent omniscience we would come to expect from God. If we are to take the formal description of the All One literally, it can be implied that the voice of God is always present, constantly repeating and speaking through the sounds and rhythms of the natural world. There is only one requirement for communing with the All One; the voice is only accessible to people who have destabilized linear perception and can parse environmental data in novel, nonlinear ways.

In accounts of mysticism and madness, God only speaks to people in states of heightened destabilization: deprivation, psychosis, schizophrenia, stress, fever, dream, trance, and hallucination. Because of this it is easy to assume that hearing the voice of God is a symptom of insanity. According to PIT, when the brain destabilizes due to hallucinogenic interrupt, it will naturally seek coherence with the strongest local periodic driver. In some cases the strongest local driver may be the shaman, it may be the jungle, it may be the refrigerator, it may be the city, it may be the croaking of frogs and crickets, it may be a jaguar stalking in the distance, it may be Gaia, or it may be God. Another way to look at it is this: God is a timeless nonlinear being; in order to hear God's voice we must be able to achieve the stillness and silence necessary to perceive and parse longitudinal nonlinear input. Without debating the metaphysical existence of God, the formal techniques for subjectively communing with the All One are reliable and repeatable, and can be readily achieved through temporary, reversible destabilization of linear perception via psychedelic drugs.

Information Capacity of Spiritual Communion

A commonly repeated theme in spiritual shamanism is that spirits are fickle and their information should not always be trusted. This is perhaps a metaphor for all psychedelic information, or information revealed in a state of nonlinear destabilization. Common sense would dictate that if spirit information is unreliable it should be uniformly discounted as delusion or insanity, but subjective reports and clinical studies show that people find great value and utility in the information generated in psychedelic experience. Common sense also dictates that the information capacity of spirit information cannot exceed the existing knowledge of the subject, but subjective reports claim that psychedelic visions reveal new wisdom all the time. The overall information value of psychedelic shamanism is thus debatable.

Since no studies exist to validate the authenticity of psychedelic spirit information, it is impossible to estimate the actual information value. From a statistical analysis we can assume that nonlinear psychedelic information emerges into consciousness at speeds far greater than linear information, generating a large pool of abstract ideas in a very short period of time. Many of the ideas generated in a psychedelic session may be delusional or fantastical, but because of the sheer volume a small percentage of them are also destined to be insightful and genius. Within the flow of psychedelic information it is up to the subject to decide which bits are useful and which bits are not, and the trick of this disambiguation comes when attempting to translate nonlinear insight to linear concepts, beliefs, and behaviors. If nonlinear insights compress easily to linear concepts, then spirit information may be of high value; if nonlinear insights are confusing or defy rationality, then perhaps the spirits are up to their old tricks again. Either way, spirit information should always be carefully parsed and analyzed for trickery and deception before being acted upon or integrated into belief.

Notes and References

1. Akers B, "The Sacred Mushrooms of Mexico: Assorted Texts". University Press of America, October 10, 2006.

2. Accounts of communing with a singular universal force under the influence of psychedelics are taken from subjective reports. Direct quotes are paraphrased.

Chapter 22

Information Genesis and Complexity

The emergence of new information over time was the obsession of psychedelic philosopher Terence McKenna, and he popularized the term Novelty Theory to describe the phenomenon of increasing information complexity in the universe through time. In order to graph the emergence of novelty through time, McKenna created an occult formula based on the hexagrams of the I Ching, and charted a jagged line that starts at zero and tops out at infinity; what he called Timewave Zero. McKenna's observation that novelty appeared to be speeding up led him to believe that time was approaching a singularity where all information tops out at infinity, set to occur on December 12, 2012.[1] The infinite complexity McKenna describes is actually the opposite of a singularity (which is zero complexity), but McKenna's observations about novelty speeding up were essentially correct. Although many people have adopted McKenna's 2012 singularity meme, the occult construction of his Timewave and other aspects of his 2012 prophecy have left many unconvinced.

Psychedelic Information Theory approaches novelty and information genesis from a different perspective than McKenna. McKenna viewed novelty as a trend line that begins with the start of the universe and speeds forward from zero until infinity, which is accurate but is also misleading at the same time. McKenna also does not differentiate between types of information and the contexts in which new information emerges; this is also a problem. By blending all information together into a single trend line, it would appear that novelty is speeding up and will soon top out at infinity, but this trend line flattens out if you consider that information exists in various states, and that each state generates information at a more or less constant rate depending on state energy density.

To illustrate the fundamentals of energy density and information complexity I have created a table that delineates the emergence of quantum levels of information systems over time, and the type of information each system generates (Table 2).

Info State	Δ^n	Time of State Change	Information Type
Singular	Δ^0	+15 billion years ago	Singularity, no information
Fundamental	Δ^1	15 billion years ago	Force breaking, strong force, electromagnetism, gravity
Luminous	Δ^2	14.99 billion years ago	Cosmic radiation, light, heat, subatomic particles
Gaseous	Δ^3	14 billion years ago	Simple atoms, hydrogen, helium, galaxy formation, stars
Elemental	Δ^4	11 billion years ago	Heavy elements, star collapse, novas, spread of heavy matter
Organic	Δ^5	4 billion years ago	Complex molecules, organic chemistry, replication, plant life
Animal	Δ^6	500-50 million years ago	Nervous systems, connective logic, memory, consciousness
Technological	Δ^7	3 million years to today	Tools, symbols, art, language, manipulation of matter and energy
Post-Tech	Δ^8	Distant future	Post-terrestrial, AI, nonlinear time and space, n dimensions

Table 2. Emergence of information systems over time: Information emerges into the universe within formal stages, each stage marking a quantum leap in energy density and the speed and complexity at which new information is produced.

Since information is created by state change over time, I have used the symbol Δ (delta, as in delta-one, delta-two, etc.) to denote stages of information creation. Each stage in the matrix represents a quantum leap in the order of energy density and complexity of information being generated, and novelty creation in the universe accelerates with each of these quantum leaps. Each stage relies on the information created in the previous state to move forward with increasing physical density and complexity. This model takes into account the Big Bang theory and the best guesses of modern astrophysics and cosmology as to when each new information level emerged, but the story of information genesis in the universe goes something like this.

Starting at Δ^0 we have the pre- Big Bang singularity where all information is condensed into a single infinitely small point. There is no state change over time, so there is no information. Around fifteen billion years ago there was a Δ^1 state change we call the Big Bang, in which the uniform singularity breaks into the fundamental forces of physics: strong nuclear force, electromagnetism, and gravity. At this stage God says "Let there be light," and we have the emergence of cosmic radiation and nuclear fusion which allows subatomic particles to form, leading to a Δ^2 state change where simple hydrogen and helium atoms can stabilize; the first matter created from condensed particles of energy. The gravity drag on this new mass allowed a Δ^3 state change where globular clouds of gasses clump and then collapsed inward, creating spinning galaxies of exploding stars fueled by nuclear fusion. When stars begin to exhaust their energy and collapse inward, there is a Δ^4 state change that allows for the creation of all the denser elements on the periodic table that can store more cosmic energy within a single point, or an atomic nucleus, which is comprised of particles of compressed energy.

The Δ^4 state represents the galactic preconditions necessary for life as we know it – the "firmament" – and in order to create the dense elements needed for life you need the fundamental forces of physics (Δ^1), an energy radiation source (Δ^2), the formation of simple gasses (Δ^3), and billions of years of nuclear fusion (Δ^4). At each stage you have a modest increase in the complexity of physical interactions which allows for new information genesis, but at the Δ^4 stage following star collapses and supernovae, we finally have the raw materials for terrestrial formation: heavy metals. A glob of heavy metal orbited our local star (the sun) and cooled to form a solid planet. As our planet cooled, liquid water formed on the surface and oxidized the metal on the outer crust, creating the nutrient-rich salt-water conditions for a Δ^5 stage change in the formation of complex molecules held together on strands of charged hydrocarbons. This marks the beginning of life.

The Δ^0 to Δ^4 information states are pre-organic and are therefore only interesting to physicists, astrophysicists, and mathematicians, but the Δ^5 information matrix is the matrix that chemists and microbiologists study; it is the study of the conditions in which energy is stored and transferred through molecular bonds. When shamen and mystics tap into the web of life and the primal force that connects all living things, they are tapping into the Δ^5 information matrix, which is sometimes described as an invisible electromagnetic field which permeates all creation, or the invisible landscape. The visual representation of this living energy field is most acute under the influence of tryptamine hallucinogens such as psilocybin and ayahuasca (DMT), and the source of this field is often perceived to be divine in origin, leading to many interesting speculations about spirit realms, Akashic fields, morphogenetic fields, and the like. Whether or not tryptamine visions are accurate representations of the electromagnetic field is a matter for some debate, but the overwhelming number of subjective accounts make the appearance of this field difficult to deny.

The Δ^5 matrix is the matrix which sustains our life; it is at work in our cellular functioning and metabolism right now. The Δ^5 matrix allows for the creation of new information at a rate that far exceeds previous information stages, and information genesis at this stage happens at the level of nucleotides, DNA, RNA, enzymes, proteins, and the organic chemistry of replication, proliferation, mutation, and Darwinian selection. Life excels at taking inert matter and organizing it into more complex forms, and in a few billion years life evolves from single-celled organisms to complex animals, representing a Δ^6 state change that allows for the development of motor nervous systems and rudimentary organism consciousness. The Δ^6 matrix relies on the Δ^5 organism matrix for cellular energy and nutritional support, but it represents a state change because the information stored in the Δ^6 matrix is neural, connective, and allows for internal storage of external state properties (or memory) at the organism level. The same connective neural network needed to control muscle behavior while navigating the external world is adapted to store memories of the external world for later use, and this internal neural storage increases organic information complexity from simple cellular organization into connective representational and symbolic logic.

The Δ^6 state change marks the most important quantum leap in the entire information chain because at Δ^6 organisms begin to internalize external data into personal connective networks. With the development of animal consciousness, the universe begins to map properties of the physical world (objective information) into connective logic stored in brains (subjective memory). Information in the Δ^6 state flows intuitively through animals in the alpha state, the tribe mind, the hive mind, and the fluid pack. The Δ^6 information matrix is semiconscious, instinctual, and routine; it is where nonverbal intuition, habitual behavior, and psychic bonding occur.

After hundreds of millions of years of animal life there is another state change brought about by evolution and morphology, the early primate adaptation of the fine finger dexterity needed to use tools. The ability for an organism to incorporate an external tool (like a rock or a stick) and a specialized skill (like throwing or pounding) into daily behavior heralded the age of technology, and with the Δ^7 state change came a corresponding shift in the speed and complexity of technological information which grows ever faster and more complex to this day. From sticks to fire to wheels and alphabets and machines and computers, hominids have excelled at incorporating information into their brains, rearranging it, and using it to externalize new information and technologies. The story of Δ^7 information genesis is the story of human culture itself, the organized spread and control of information through hominid tribal groups leading to power, civilization, empire, and industry.

The Δ^7 information matrix represents another quantum leap in information genesis, storage, and transmission. The logic networks created by internalizing reality in the neural Δ^6 matrix are used to create new information which is externalized in the form of technology, language, art, media, and invention. The Δ^7 information state is the realm of language, logic, critical thinking, science, and rational analysis. Modern culture cherishes the Δ^7 information space above all others, this is the space where the tools of mythology, religion, politics, and mathematics emerge. The Δ^7 information space occupies an ego-driven, distracted, beta state of critical self-awareness. Like charged particles seeking to find electromagnetic balance, the human in the Δ^7 state will seek to correct or improve perceived problems with external reality via subjectively controlled ingenuity. Total mastery over the subjective manipulation of matter and energy is the ultimate goal of the Δ^7 information state, the state humans have almost perfected. Now that we have the internet, supercolliders, nanotech, and atomic bombs, all of these technologies seem to herald another quantum information state change in the near future.

The Singularity and Post-Technological Matrices

The Δ^8 information state can be called the post-technology state, and much like McKenna's Timewave Zero, the technological Δ^7 information matrix must eventually top out with the end of science and the complete integration of all physical forces into human technology. This seems like it is happening quickly, but going by trends in previous state changes the singularity isn't likely to happen for another few-hundred-thousand to a million years from now. Though it is currently impossible to imagine what a Δ^8 information space might be like, subjective control over the very fabric of space and time may become possible, allowing something like personal access to space travel, time travel, alternate time streams, and/or an infinite number of parallel dimensions. From the perspective of a Δ^7 information state, a Δ^8 state change would look like subjective human information topping out at infinity; Δ^8 consciousness will have instant access to everything there is to know about humans, technology, the universe, and whatever lies beyond. I believe this Δ^8 state transition is what McKenna perceived in his novelty wave as the end of information.

If we are to follow the permutations of information complexity to date, it is logical to assume that the technology created in the Δ^7 matrix will directly contribute to the fundamental state variables needed for a Δ^8 state change. This can be interpreted to mean that machine code is the next level of information energy density and computers will drive complexity and information genesis into the Δ^8 state. Perhaps this transition is already underway, and is approaching a quantum leap in technology where computers begin generating information and complexity for their own purposes. Only time will tell if this is the case, but in a few hundred thousand years it is conceivable that machine intelligence will be ubiquitous throughout the galaxy, and the end-point of our technology will become the initial conditions needed for the evolution of a more durable and complex matrix.

Shamanism and Information Matrices

When a shaman enters the trance state and searches for new information, there are specific levels of knowledge which are more helpful than others. For instance, when entering group mind with the tribe, the shaman will want to access a pre-technology Δ^6 information matrix where primal animal consciousness, non-verbal communication, and pack bonding instincts are strongest. If the shaman wants to commune with plant intelligence he will enter into a Δ^5 matrix of cellular metabolism and genetic expression; this is also where the shaman will diagnose disease and attempt healing by visualizing and diverting the flow of metabolic energy through the patient's cells with bodywork and sound. Some shaman may also commune with the more cosmic levels of awareness, but shamanism is essentially a Δ^7 technology used by Δ^6 organisms to access information available in Δ^{0-5} matrices; information which is always present but is normally invisible or beyond the limits of human perception.

Notes and References

1. McKenna T, "The Invisible Landscape". Harper, San Francisco, 1993.

Appendix 01

Conclusions and Discussion

Conclusions

The primary tenets of Psychedelic Information Theory dictate that hallucinogens generate information by destabilizing linear perception to promote nonlinear states of consciousness; that these states amplify initial conditions provided by set and setting; that these states increase in nonlinear complexity in response to dose of hallucinogen, duration of effect, and strength of sensory stimulation; and that the depth or complexity of psychedelic hallucination can be controlled through pitch-timed, rhythmic, or periodic sensory feedback stimulation.

The tenets of the Control Interrupt Model dictate that top-down feedback control of multisensory perception must be destabilized before consciousness can bifurcate, become nonlinear, and generate hallucination; that the destabilizing interrupt of any hallucinogen can be felt subjectively as a periodic pulsation or interference pattern in the range of human sensory temporal aliasing; that sensory complexity or animated progression of hallucination iterates along the frequency of the periodic interrupt; that each hallucinogen has a distinct sensory interrupt frequency and ADSR envelope based on its affinity and selective agonism in sensory binding pathways; and that the unique interrupt and ADSR envelope created by each molecule is responsible for its unique hallucinogenic patterns and multisensory signatures.

The tenets of Shamanism in the Age of Reason, or Physical Shamanism, dictate that a shaman can intuitively sense the interrupt frequency and ADSR envelope of any hallucinogen simply by ingesting a small amount of the substance and paying close attention to the interference patterns created in perception; that shamanic *icaros* or standing vocalizations use harmonic interference to drive or dampen the amplitude of hallucinogenic interrupt; that driving the amplitude of hallucinogenic interrupt increases depth of iteration and complexity in nonlinear information organization; that shamanic dieting and purging is a precursor to destabilizing metabolic homeostasis necessary for holistic nonlinear re-modulation; that bodily transcendence relies on full nonlinear amplification along all cellular signaling pathways, from the gut to the cortex; and that full nonlinear breakthroughs, or psychedelic peak experiences, are only achieved once top-down homeostasis is fully interrupted and the subject releases all inhibitory feedback control over the resulting emergent process.

The basic conclusions taken from the tenets of Psychedelic Information Theory, the Control Interrupt Model, and Physical Shamanism are as follows.

1. Psychedelics generate information in the human organism via nonlinear feedback amplification of both intercellular (neural) and intracellular (cytoplasmic) signaling mechanisms.

2. The nonlinear amplification of sensation exploits excitatory feedback mechanisms used to create lasting emotional attachments to salient sensory patterns in the wake of strong incoming stimulus.

3. Psychedelic hallucination and expanded states of consciousness represent nonlinear amplification of initial conditions of biology, perception, memory, behavior, and location, otherwise known as set and setting.

4. Nonlinear amplification of sensation promotes neuroplasticity and cellular regeneration via hormonal and stress-based mechanisms related to cell proliferation and long-term memory consolidation.

5. Periods of chaotic transition between multi-stable states of consciousness are subjectively perceived as disorienting, confusing, and uncomfortable. Periods where chaotic transitions approach strange attractors and phase-lock into multi-stability

are subjectively perceived as ecstatic, beautiful, spiritual, insightful, cleansing, healing, and transcendent.

6. Extended periods of iterating complexity in cellular networks leads to states of consciousness perceived as enlightening, mystical, infinite, god-like, timeless, Gnostic, and omniscient.

7. Resistance to nonlinear destabilization under the influence of psychedelics results in anxiety spirals, panic, and potentially paranoid and psychotic states.

8. There is an optimal dose range for any hallucinogen where states of nonlinear organization and strange attractors spontaneously emerge. Moving beyond the optimal dose range results in highly unpredictable, uncontrollable, and problematic states of consciousness resembling psychosis and schizophrenia.

9. States of nonlinear organization in neural networks can be stabilized through energetic periodic drivers, such as music, singing, chanting, and dancing; making psychedelic consciousness multi-stable along a range of complex output.

10. Through entrainment and mutual feedback, nonlinear states of cellular signaling can transcend individuals to promote pack mind, group mind, peer bonding, mate bonding, and spontaneous nonverbal organization of tribal or familial structures.

11. Shamanic healing, entheogenic transcendence, and psychedelic creativity all utilize nonlinear amplification to generate novelty in the form of spontaneous energetic organization in cellular signaling systems.

12. Because psychedelics produce uniquely nonlinear states of consciousness, any art which evokes recurrence, chaos, and nonlinear forms will be immediately recognizable as psychedelic.

13. Nonlinear forms are perceived to be inherently beautiful and spiritual because they are isomorphic of ordered complexity in the generative processes of biology and nature; thus psychedelic hallucination is perceived as inherently beautiful and spiritual.

Discussion

The fundamentals of PIT were assembled through formal analysis of hallucinogenic states, shamanic ritual, and subjective reports of expanded consciousness. PIT is a general theory, which means it seeks to model an approximation of psychedelic information complexity emerging into human consciousness and cultural memory. PIT applies existing physical models and mathematical concepts like wave mechanics, coupled oscillators, and deterministic chaos to the processes of perception and consciousness. Some components of PIT's general theory can be easily modeled with mathematical or mechanical counterparts; other components are assumed or presumed from observation and published research; and other components are pure speculation or are left purposely vague due to lack of proper corroborating research. Some of these assumptions, speculations, and missing pieces are discussed here.

First and foremost, PIT assumes that the human brain acts as a resonant oscillator, and that consciousness is the result of time-synchronized interference patterns of recurrent neural spike trains cascading through the neocortex. This is not a radical model, it is based on the fundamentals of neural oscillators, periodic drivers, wave entrainment, resonance, and coherence. Entrainment is the capacity for one oscillator to synchronize the frequency of a group of oscillators; resonance is the capacity for one oscillator to drive the amplitude of another oscillator; coherence is when two oscillators phase-lock into stable resonant or harmonic interference patterns to conserve or amplify energy. Classical wave mechanics and the behaviors of feedback coupled harmonic oscillators are the starting point for almost every new concept introduced in PIT.

The Control Interrupt Model and Physical Shamanism both invoke resonant wave interference as a means of producing coherent patterns of nonlinear organization in oscillating systems. Using sound or vibration to produce spontaneous organization of matter is also known as cymatics, which can be demonstrated with sand on a vibrating steel plate. As the steel plate vibrates at various resonant frequencies, the sand will spontaneously move from chaotic to organized patterns, also known as Chladni patterns or nodal patterns (Fig. 31). Cymatics is an example of oscillating systems finding stability at normal modes. Modal vibration can be characterized by period doubling or halving a system's fundamental frequency to create harmonic interference at one of many possible resonant frequencies. This is a mathematical concept that applies to music, coupled oscillators, modal theory, quantum theory, standing waves, and so on.

Analyzing the brain, perception, and consciousness as a single standing wave or resonant oscillator is a very crude simplification of much more complex sensory process, but the general models of feedback control, destabilization, and chaos apply universally in all oscillating systems. Framing the discussion of psychedelics and shamanism in terms of the nonlinear dynamics of resonant oscillators may not shine light on the entire psychedelic experience, but it provides a comprehensive and succinct formal approximation of perceptual complexity generated in expanded states of consciousness, which is the ultimate goal of PIT.

By invoking stability and chaos in perceptual networks, PIT also assumes there are specific organized-chaotic states of psychedelic consciousness that act as strange attractors to pull perception towards multi-stable convergence points. PIT also implies that resonant periodic drivers, such as shamanic singing or drumming, can entrain, stabilize, and amplify convergent multi-stable psychedelic states, or equilibrium states, to induce healing, transcendence, and group mind. However, PIT offers no specific descriptions of precise shamanic frequencies or equilibrium states as practical evidence of this theory. Because the published research in the field of psychedelic brain scanning is limited, the assertions of shamanic entrainment and multi-state phase locking are speculative and based solely on subjective reports and observation of the dynamics of shamanic ritual. PIT provides no formal definition for what a multi-stable psychedelic state looks like on a scanning device compared to a normal state of consciousness, nor does it say where or how one should scan for the best statistical indicators of such states. This is an issue that can only be resolved through statistical analysis of many controlled psychedelic scanning sessions in the presence of live music or shamanic ceremony compared against sessions of meditation or trance dancing. It may be decades before such research becomes available, and even when it is available there is no guarantee it will be conclusive enough to distinctly target specific mystical states.

Because psychedelics are non-specific amplifiers and can produce multiple outcomes based on initial conditions of dose, set, and setting, the concept of scanning brains to provide a single unified definition of an expanded state of consciousness may be inherently flawed. Psychedelics can induce trance, catatonia, hallucination, psychosis, paranoia, mania, hysteria, and euphoria all in response to unobservable conditions in dose, set, and setting, so they are demonstrably capable of inducing many complex states of altered consciousness. Psychedelic amplification of perception is observably nonlinear in the form of fractal hallucinations, and the nonlinear amplification of perception is observably tied to size of dose of hallucinogen and strength of incoming stimulus. A model where strong sensory drivers can entrain multi-stable states of nonlinear psychedelic consciousness is a small extrapolation of these simple observations. Technically, any song or chant produced by a shaman should entrain an organized psychedelic state along a range of chaotic, stable, and multi-stable output. Studying the biofeedback equilibrium effects of spontaneous shamanic vocalization (*icaros*) in a live group setting may be the best starting place for examining tones and frequencies for driving attractor states for each hallucinogen at each dose range. Isolating which songs are best for producing which states at which dose range may ultimately be more of an art than science, relying less on statistical research and more on the shaman's intuitive grasp of all the sliding state variables unique to each psychedelic session.

The conclusion of PIT is that attractors, or multi-stable convergence points in expanded consciousness, do exist, that they are physical in nature, and that when a subject locks into these states they are nothing less than magical. Finding the sweet spots in neural oscillator coherence where consciousness diverges and becomes exponentially complex may be elusive, or may involve different indicators for each individual. General nonlinear dynamics suggests that expanded states of consciousness may be achieved by entraining limit cycles of perception into period doubled bifurcations of normal output, with each period-doubling preceded by some critical sensory stimulus or spiking activity required to drive the phase transition. This driving action also describes the dynamics of entraining stable or self-sustaining limit cycles in a forced Van der Pol oscillator, which is one of the simplest and earliest demonstrations of deterministic chaos in physical systems. Although first applied to electrical circuits, the Van der Pol equation can also be applied to social and theoretical constructs, like species reproduction or the dynamic effects of repetitive marketing on brand goodwill. Mode locking into period doubled or reverse period doubled stability is the general model of state bifurcation in dynamical systems (Fig. 30), though applying a simple nonlinear circuit model to perception raises some processing questions. If perception can jump limit cycles and bifurcate into analyzing multiple simultaneous frames along the order of 3-to-4 times, moving from aliasing 2 frames to 4, and then to 8, and then to 16 simultaneous frames, where does the extra frame aliasing power come from?

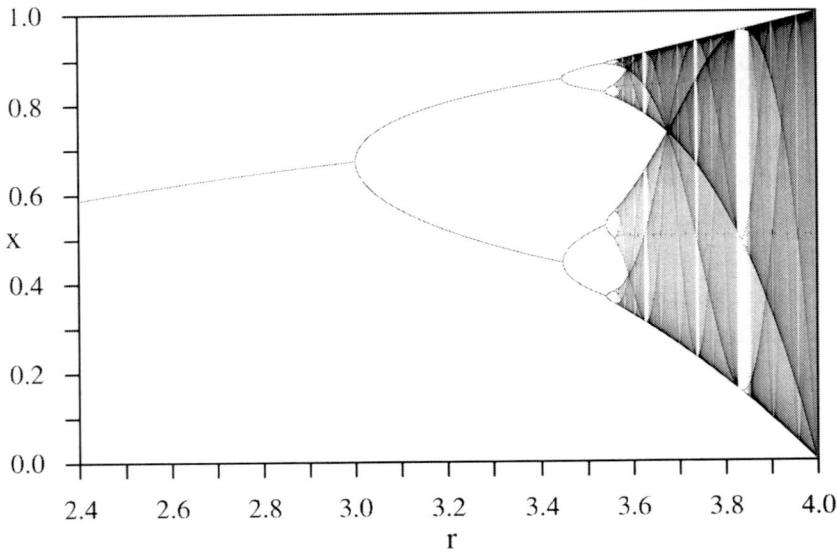

Figure 30. Period doubling bifurcations in the logistics map $x_{n+1} = rx_n(1 - x_n)$. The form recedes with self similarity as periods of chaos are followed by periods of convergence and stability. From WikiPedia, Bifurcation Diagram.

The Frame Stacking Model assumes that periodic doubling of frame complexity does not necessarily require a full linear doubling of energy input, but is instead is the result of iterated mapping, or nonlinear feedback amplification driving novel re-organization, or phase transitions, through states of chaotic interference and harmonic convergence. For instance, a video camera falling into a chaotic feedback loop does not require extra energy for the transition to stacking multiple receding frames, but the feedback process quickly overwhelms the camera's detail rendering as receding frames over 16 layers deep begin to smooth together in stable interference patterns, or strange attractors, converging on archetypal images of fractal curves, kaleidoscopes, concentric mandalas, galactic vortexes, infinite tunnels, DNA spirals, ascending staircases, and so on (Fig. 24).

Where and how these nonlinear phase transitions occur in human consciousness is still a matter for some speculation. The best evidence indicates that psychedelics promote sensory saturation at the apical dendrite columns of the neocortex, leading to destabilization in recurrent thalamocortical and corticocortical binding pathways. Frame stacking may also be related to receding frame detail being sustained and looped through recurrent circuits between the PFC, basal forebrain, and midbrain. Delaying neutralization or period-doubling saturation intensity in these recurrent mid-brain circuits could lead to frame-feedback or sustained frame echo with high perceived salience. It may seem logical that psychedelic action is localized in the brain, but given the distribution of 5-HT receptors and the indiscriminate nature of ligand binding, it is reasonable to assume that psychedelic amplification in cellular signaling networks is both global and globally coherent. Tracking the physiology of temporal frame aliasing, frame neutralization, frame repetition, and how these sensory mechanisms are exploited by working memory, learning, dreaming, and psychedelics is an area ripe for further exploration.

Finally, the frame model of perception forwarded in PIT is only an approximation of actual perception. While the frame model allows us to put a distinct limit on the rate of human temporal aliasing (roughly 15 frames per second), there is evidence that humans can track multiple moving layers in any single frame. Instead of updating in perfect frames like a film reel, perception is more like a compressed MPEG video or an animation that updates a full keyframe whenever the eyes blink or move, and only makes minor layering changes in between each keyframe. For instance, if you are standing in a grassy meadow watching a bird fly through the air, your brain does not need to update the entire frame of the meadow to track the bird, it only needs to update the layer with the motion of the bird. In this way the brain conserves energy and saves state information for those areas that do not need constant updating, and only updates the entire multisensory frame every few seconds or so, such as when you blink or shift your focus. This motion-sensitive updating of non-essential background noise is most evident in Troxler's fading illusion (Fig. 5).

Tracking multiple layers for each frame adds another level of complexity to the simplified Frame Stacking Model, and may suggest how psychedelic perception can become kaleidoscopic as radial sections in the visual field mirror themselves, stack, drift, and merge together. Because the update and release of perceptual layers in both multi-layered or radial frame filling methods still falls under the classification of temporal aliasing and filling, the general models of PIT would still apply regardless of the morphological or geometric nature of the perceptual bifurcation. The Control Interrupt and Frame Stacking models are provided as very general meta-level descriptions of how psychedelics may subvert temporal aliasing and filling to produce nonlinear feedback and self-sustaining hallucination. While PIT has been focused primarily on visual sensory networks, these models can be applied to the layering and splintering of any subjective sensation of self or reality. The specific pharmacological and neural models underlying these general concepts are more complex than can be detailed in this text, but are sufficiently well understood to make good approximations supporting PIT's claims. Since PIT was designed to be general theory, even as our understanding of perception and pharmacology changes, the general assumptions forwarded here should still apply to all known types of hallucinogenic experience.

Appendix 02

Informal Discussion of Topics

The following is an interview-style discussion of topics presented in *Psychedelic Information Theory* with the author, provided as a summary and general overview of theory for the non-scientific layperson.

What is Psychedelic Information Theory?

The general theory underlying all of PIT is that psychedelics create information when introduced to human neural networks. The spontaneous creation of new information is the essential function of psychedelic activation, and this new information is imprinted into memory and reproduced as music, art, or stories shared with other people. More specifically, PIT presents physical models which describe this generative process, and the dynamics of various psychedelic phenomena like complex hallucination, shamanism, and group mind.

How does PIT describe psychedelic action?

One way to visualize what I'm describing in PIT is through what I call the "Pond and the Pump House" metaphor. Imagine a perfectly round pond with perfectly still water, with a small pump house sitting on an island in the center. When the pump house is turned on it sends out perfectly circular ripples through the water that, over time, create a neatly ordered standing wave of activity. In this metaphor the pond is the surface of the neocortex; the pump house is the body, heartbeat, and respiration; and the ripples are waves of sensory perception seen in an EEG reading of cortical activity. When the pump is on and moving at different speeds, the ripples on the surface of the pond are active and take on different coherent patterns; when the pump is turned off the ripples fade and the pond becomes still and quiet. These are metaphors for consciousness moving from waking to sleeping states.

Now imagine we add a psychedelic to this model. PIT proposes that psychedelics alter the wave patterns of consciousness by creating a tiny tremor under the pond that vibrates the entire structure. Adding the psychedelic to the system creates a competing standing wave that can be seen immediately in the ripples on the surface. The pump keeps pumping, creating its usual standing waves, but because of the tremor there is a new layer of complexity to the ripple patterns. The tremor adds energy to the system, and as it does the standing waves in the pond become more chaotic. Instead of simple coherent ripple patterns, you begin to see overlapping patterns and fast transitions between multiple standing wave states. The complex interference patterns overlap on themselves and exhibit the formal qualities of nonlinear feedback system, such as fractals or cellular automata.

The interference pattern in the ripples of the pond described here is how PIT models a competing tryptamine agonist (a hallucinogen) in the finely timed aminergic system of perception, modulated by serotonin and dopamine. This complex interference pattern is what I am describing with the Control Interrupt Model of psychedelic action. According to PIT, each hallucinogen creates a slightly different tremor or vibration in the signaling pathways of multisensory awareness, which in-turn creates a unique and distinct interference pattern in the standing waves of perception. Some hallucinogenic tremors may be big and rolling, others may be quiet and subtle, others may be sharp and disruptive. The difference in tremor speed and feel created by each psychedelic molecule would be accounted for by the differing receptor affinities and metabolic pathways for each hallucinogen.

How do psychedelic interference patterns relate to the techniques of shamanism and psychedelic therapy?

Let's go back to our pond metaphor. Assume there are sand dunes created at the edges of the pond that correspond to the long-term memory of the standing wave patterns created by the pump house. If you check these dunes after each psychedelic tremor you might find new tiny fractals, spirals, curves, cracks, and filigreed patterns etched into the sand. These sand etchings correspond to the memory of the psychedelic experience now embedded in the patterns of the neural network, and these memory patterns then inform behavior, change beliefs, and are presented over and over again in art, music, and philosophy. That is a metaphor for transformative psychedelic therapy.

Now let's assume there is a tribe of people living at the shores of this pond, and this psychedelic tremor hits once a week. It would be perfectly reasonable to assume that these people would adopt the psychedelic sand patterns as a kind of tribal identity, and embed those patterns into their clothes, tattoos, face paints, pottery, and so on. This is exactly what tribes who take psychedelics do; they embed the colorful fractal patterns created on the surface of their brains onto the surfaces of their bodies, their artwork, their walls, and their world. The physical spilling over of complex psychedelic patterns from a single underlying ripple effect is the foundation of PIT. Psychedelic Information Theory studies the movement of complex information from the genesis of initial hallucinogenic interference pattern to the outward organizing effect on belief, personality, behavior, and tribal structure.

Now, to go one step further, assume that whenever the psychedelic tremor strikes, the tribe of people living at the shores all gather in a circle and begin to sing, or stamp their feet, or beat large drums in unison. The songs produced by the tribe will naturally fall into harmony with the tremor and begin to shape the ripples in the pond through harmonic interference. Over time, if the tribe sings loud enough, they will produce a standing interference pattern, or group hallucination, in the ripples of the pond. This can be described as a shared state of consciousness locked through a standing resonant feedback wave. Shaping interference patterns in consciousness through singing or resonant feedback describes the basic ritual techniques of psychedelic shamanism. Through resonant feedback the shaman and the tribe can master the nonlinear dynamics of the interference pattern to work various forms of magic on the surface of the pond.

The Control Interrupt Model reduces hallucinogenic action to a high speed sensory attack and decay envelope. Why did you decide on that model?

While studying the effects of various hallucinogens, I would always notice a carrier wave, or a high-pitched frequency, or a pulsing, or a throbbing, or a tingling, or some kind of stable interference that was familiar to that substance. And after studying various trip reports for various substances, I realized I was not alone in recording these simple observations. This stable interference is often reported to permeate all sensation; touch, hearing, vision, the entire body. I began to measure the frequencies of these pulses and tingles for different hallucinogens and realized that they all fell into alpha and beta states of consciousness, between 4 to 30 pulses per second, and each drug had a slightly different timing and feel to the way the pulses came on and interrupted consciousness. The slower the interruption, the more of a throbbing or stuttering I felt; the faster the interruption, the more of a tingling, vibration, or high-pitched tremor I felt.

At some point in my analysis of different drugs, I would always say, "That stable interrupt frequency is interesting, I should take a closer look at that," or, "Isn't it weird that I always feel this throbbing on this specific drug, which feels very similar to the pulsing I noticed on this other drug." And then as I began analyzing that one simple pulse interaction, I wondered if pulse interruption in frame perception was all that was needed to produce hallucination. Mind machines produce phosphenes within a small range of light pulse frequencies, so what if hallucinogens did something similar in the same pulse range? What if those pulses were the drug's only action, and the throbbing was the perceptual aggregate of modulatory interference at sensory binding junctions? During the process of formally describing the action of these pulses, it became obvious that the pulsing interference was a carrier wave for hallucination, like the flickering frame rate of an animation reel. The pulses created an overlapping hallucinogenic flicker, or an overlapping modulatory ripple, in multisensory awareness, that creates the chaotic substrate for complex hallucination. It was an extrapolation of psychedelic pharmacology that scaled up to make sense in gross perception, which was the exact kind of model I was looking for.

The more I analyzed the various properties of the flicker or pulsation for each drug, the more I realized that this specific pulsing function was the thing that caused each drug to produce unique geometric hallucinations, like Chladi forms taking on different standing wave patterns on steel plates resonating at different frequencies. I then realized that each hallucinogen could be modeled with a unique interrupt frequency and properties of saturation attack, decay, sustain, and release (ADSR) to describe the onset and feel of distinct hallucinations. An ADSR envelope is a wave modeling technique used in electronic synthesizers to shape the tones and sounds of various musical instruments, but can be used to model the "voice" for any standing wave. The ADSR envelope for each hallucinogen corresponds to receptor agonism and affinity, which naturally shapes the tone and feel of each hallucinogen's unique sensory patterns. After reducing hallucinogenic action to a function of wave interference in perception, it was then only natural to extrapolate hallucination as a cascading event that starts with a small, stable, perturbation in perceptual feedback that grows in amplitude over time to entrain the functional output of the entire system. This model does not rely on anything other than targeted receptor agonism to drive the resulting emergent process.

Why is a wave model of psychedelic action better than traditional shamanic models?

One of the core concepts of physics and science is that every physical interaction can be modeled in discrete packets of energy transfer, and these discrete packets can be statistically interpreted as waves that have formal characteristics of amplitude, frequency, coherence, decay, and so on. This allows a system to be described by predictive physical or mathematical models. Once you break any physical interaction down to a formal wave model, you've essentially described the functionality of the system and can make accurate predictions. Traditional shamanic models are not interested in this level of reductive analysis, but modern science is. PIT fills in some of the formal pieces needed to place techniques of traditional shamanism within the domains of physics and mathematics.

Doesn't reductive analysis take the mystery or artistry out of entheogenic transcendence and shamanism?

There has been a schism in shamanic thought where the drugs have been studied with a reductive pharmacological paradigm, yet the technology of shamanism is still stuck in anthropological or spiritual paradigms. What I am trying to say with PIT is that there is no schism; psychedelic action and shamanism are both fields of physics, they can both be described by physics. This is not a reductive model, it is a unifying model that knits the fields of pharmacology and shamanism together through classical wave mechanics and harmonic theory.

A similar way to look at it might be this. Imagine you were a guitar maker, and you knew precisely how long the neck of the guitar should be, and how tight each string must be, and where each fret must go, and what shape the body should be, all to produce the best and most resonant musical sound. This is an engineering task that can be described by mathematics and harmonic wave theory. However, picking up the instrument and using it to play music that moves people to joy or tears is a process will always be mysterious and artistic. Nothing has been taken away from the artistry of the musician by describing the harmonic theory at the foundation of the instrument. If anything, the harmonic theory allows the guitar maker to produce a better instrument and the musician to attain better mastery.

How do psi phenomenon like telepathy and group mind tie into PIT's harmonic wave model?

You can think of non-verbal communication betweens tribes of humans in terms of group coherence, like the swarming of insects, schooling of fish, or flocking of birds. For most daily interactions we keep ourselves separated as individuals, but for certain activities we drop into a cooperative mode where identity is less important than fluid or harmonic movement within the pack. In humans this can be seen in team sports like soccer or basketball, in the coordinated movements of military squads, in group dancing, or in the intuitive rhythms of lovemaking. Locking into harmonic coherence with another human or group of humans is subjectively felt as nonverbal communication or psi, sometimes reaching the level of telepathy, or instantly knowing what the other person is thinking. Again, this kind of process should not be analyzed within the fields of parapsychology or mysticism. When you're talking about psi and nonverbal communication, you are talking about synchrony and entrainment between resonant oscillators. That is not metaphysics, it is harmonic theory and physics.

Can you describe a resonant oscillator? How does harmonic resonance apply to the brain?

An oscillator is just another term for a wave or vibration, so any system that has a cycling frequency, which is just about everything, is an oscillator. When two oscillators near each other are vibrating near the same frequency they begin to have overlapping wave patterns, or interference patterns, that can be modeled in terms of complimentary synchrony, harmony, phase differentials, and so on. If two oscillators have complimentary interference patterns they are said to be harmonic, meaning they do not dampen each other's power or amplitude. If the two oscillators interfere in a way that drives both of their amplitudes, maximizing the potential energy of the circuit, then they are said to be in resonant coherence. When an oscillating system phase-locks into resonant coherence with another oscillator, energy is amplified and the phase-locked system becomes self-stabilizing and difficult to dampen or perturb even with a competing interference wave.

Harmonic and resonant feedback are at the center of all self-stabilizing oscillating systems, or self-oscillators. Harmonic wave interference conserves energy and is perceived as beautiful to humans in both the arts and the sciences. Loss of harmonic feedback in coupled oscillators drives chaos and chaotic output; resonant feedback and entrainment creates stable attractors and convergence in chaotic systems. These are the fundamentals of all physical systems that oscillate and trade energy over time. If you examine EEG readings it is obvious that the brain is an oscillator with distinct wave patterns for each state of consciousness, and each neuron is a tiny oscillator passing waves of information through an intricately coupled network. So applying the dynamics of resonant oscillators and harmonic wave interference to human perception and expanded states of consciousness is not a radical or fringe idea, it is a natural extension of existing physical theory.

So shamanic singing is a form of resonant feedback for stabilizing consciousness in chaotic psychedelic states?

That is the theory of Physical Shamanism in a nutshell. If you can understand that you can understand almost everything I am modeling with PIT. The interaction starts at the cellular level with a simple pharmacological interference pattern, then erupts into a chaotic ripple across the surface of the neocortex, which then bleeds over into long term memory, informs behavioral changes, and ultimately affects the values of the larger tribe and culture. The chaotic, high-information ripple extends outward over time and goes beyond the confines of the user's mind, expanding into art and media and science and religion and cultural trends. I don't think anyone has ever attempted to deconstruct the entire psychedelic information chain before, let alone attempt to fit it into some kind of physical theory. It is totally new territory.

Clearly, when someone discovers the psychedelic experience they do not keep it to themselves. There is an inherent need to change behaviors and share the experience with others, and that shared experience bounces around the culture and creates resonant interference patterns with shared artwork and reports from other psychedelic experiences, and the amount of detail and spontaneous cultural and tribal organization emerging from this process is enormous. When you attempt to model the psychedelic process with some kind of longitudinal cultural analysis, you see we are dealing with a self-sustaining nonlinear information system that is feeding back on itself through time and producing a disproportionately large amount of output in response to a very small amount of input, which is literally a single pinch of white powder per subject. Somehow, adding that little pinch of white powder ends up changing the world.

Does PIT present a hallucinogenic scale, like the Shulgin scale, which rates hallucination or expanded consciousness along some metric?

The Frame Stacking Model describes degrees of depth and complexity to hallucination, and proposes that depth of hallucination is equal to potency of substance times dose of substance, saturating and feeding back on itself over duration of effect (which is the nonlinear component), modified by the rate of metabolism for that substance. You could write this description as a mathematical formula, but what it is attempting to explain is that there is a critical dose range for each drug where the depth of hallucination becomes self-sustaining and naturally drives towards a fully animated frame rate of about 8-16 stacked frames per second, like an attractor pulling you towards a "peaking" state. If the dose of psychedelic is too small or you metabolize it too quickly, you only get a slightly speedy or jittery sensation corresponding to interference in perception; no peaking state. But once you find the right dose range and achieve self-sustaining hallucination, you lock into this expanded state where you begin stacking progressively animated frames until you top out around 16 receding frames deep. Anything over 16 stacked frames of temporal depth converges towards infinity and overwhelms human perception.

You could break the Shulgin scale down by depth of hallucinogenic frame complexity if you wanted to, but the model PIT suggests is very generic, like a screen saver algorithm or stacked video feedback loop. The Shulgin scale does not attempt to model this kind of complexity in hallucination, nor should it. PIT is attempting to model a more granular level of sensory detail.

You say expanded consciousness tops out at 16 stacked frames? Why 16 frames?

The number 16 seems a bit arbitrary, but it was the number proposed by the person who first described the Frame Stacking Model to me, and this frame depth was upheld to some degree by my own experimentation with mechanical video feedback as well as a variety of hallucinogenic substances. The frame stacking model is an attempt to quantify the fast rate of progressive animation created by hallucination, and to formalize the rate at which sensation saturates, echoes, stacks, regresses, smears, or overlaps into the subsequent perceptual frame. This is a morphological approach to studying the dynamics of progressive hallucination, and you can measure the liquidity or stretchiness of any hallucination based on this metric of seamless smoothing or aliasing between overlapping stacked frames. After about 16 frames of depth, things tend to trail off and blur together into infinitely receding mist.

With the frame stacking model you can step back and analyze your own hallucination and ask; is it flickering and pulsing like a strobe light, or is it oozing slowly with a high degree of fine detail? The more motion trails you are seeing, the more echoes you're hearing, the more liquid and fluid the hallucination seems, all of that corresponds to the number of simultaneous frames you are stacking. After about 16 layers of temporal frame regression, perception begins to saturate and melt and converge down this white spiral or tunnel into infinity. Experiencing this vortex or tunnel, like your mind being sucked out of your body, is a common sensation on large doses of psychedelics. It may be called ego death, or peaking, or whiting out, or a near-death experience, but it is very much like passing out and going unconscious and leaving your body. It is nearly impossible to have any control over thought, action, memory, or behavior past this perceptual capacity. At this point most people lie down and go astral.

How do you think PIT will be perceived in the future?

Most psychedelic theory is built around cultural notions of self and spirituality, and because of this most theories typically have a shelf-life of a few decades. Instead of using metaphors, PIT was built around physical models and the best understanding of the physiology of the brain and perception. This gives PIT a much longer shelf-life than previous psychedelic theory. And since PIT avoids spiritual metaphor it is also applicable across all cultures. PIT is not the final word in the field of psychedelic shamanism, but it provides a neat general framework for the study of expanded consciousness. It is my hope that future generations of explorers will read this text and be inspired to evaluate psychedelic phenomena with a more critical scientific eye.

What experiments can be done to test the various models presented in PIT?

PIT is already a working theory. The process and outcomes of shamanism and psychedelic experimentation have already been formalized and tested. Further testing cannot disprove PIT, but it can help refine the level of detail in the proposed models. PIT was informed by existing research from hundreds if not thousands of different sources, including both published scientific literature, traditional shamanic ritual, and underground research from anonymous psychedelic explorers. PIT does not seek to undo research or suggest further avenues for research, but instead proposes a physical model that can tie all existing research together.

All of the models proposed by PIT come directly from studying subjective reports of psychedelic experience and shamanic ritual, and then overlaying these reports with the most current research on psychedelic receptor interaction along various perceptual pathways. All of the models, methods, and techniques described in PIT have been tested in humans and are accurate. Shamanism is already in common practice with only crude spirit models or psychological models to work with. The only thing left to do is refine our understanding of the brain, and as our understanding grows we can look back at the existing shamanic model and ask, "Is it still accurate?" And if the answer is no, then we need to refine the model and make it more accurate. That's the ongoing labor of science.

About this Text

About Psychedelic Information Theory

Psychedelic Information Theory (PIT) began in 2004 as an extended essay entitled "The Case Against DMT Elves," which was a response to a web article entitled "DMT, Moses, and the Quest for Transcendence" by Clifford Pickover. "The Case Against DMT Elves" was meant to be an antithesis to the "spirit world" models of DMT popularized by Terence McKenna and Rick Strassman in the 1990s, and as such it received some support for taking a more formal approach to examining hallucination. When I realized that the physiological case for complex hallucination had never been sufficiently compiled, I collected some notes and previous writings and began to assemble the PIT Alpha version on the tripzine.com website, which also includes an archive of material from *Trip Magazine*, a journal of psychedelic culture which I published from 1995 through 2005.

The process of putting the PIT Alpha version together took over a year and included the help of many people sending donations, proofreading, and providing valuable feedback on the text. PIT Alpha began as an attempt to reduce psychedelic phenomenology from a purely connective and pharmacological perspective. Sometime in late 2005, halfway through the text of PIT Alpha, I completely abandoned this approach. In 2006 I adopted a circuit model of psychedelic activation I dubbed Signal Theory, which emphasized the role of recurrent excitation in cortical networks as the source of hallucinogenesis. A summary of this theory was presented at the 2006 *Toward a Science of Consciousness* conference in Tucson, AZ. Over a period of two years Signal Theory evolved into what I called the Multi-State Theory of psychedelic action, which was the first time I considered the full implications of psychedelics as catalysts for multi-stable states of nonlinear consciousness.

After releasing a review version of the Multi-State Theory online, I received some interesting feedback that helped focus my thinking, some of it coming from an anonymous Canadian researcher who shared his unique theory of hallucinogenic frame stacking to simplify my theory of recurrent feedback. This led me to study the various nonlinear effects produced by a competing modulator in a precisely timed sequential frame processing system. By extrapolating the various overlapping pharmacological, circuit, and network models of psychedelic action, I settled upon the Control Interrupt Model, which posits that all hallucination begins with a high-frequency periodic interruption of multisensory frame stability that could be described as a wave interference pattern. Once the Control Interrupt Model fell into place, Psychedelic Information Theory suddenly made sense again, and the entire text was rewritten from this new perspective.

After the six year effort on this project, I can proudly say that PIT is the model of hallucinogenesis and psychedelic action I was always seeking to produce. I believe PIT sheds a unique light on the processes of human consciousness and the capacity of the human imagination, and will serve psychedelic research and altered-state exploration for many years. I sincerely thank all of the people who sent donations, feedback, and subtle reminders over the years. Many thanks to all the people who followed my work and kept me focused on finishing, I could not have done it without the consistent support encouragement.

Sincerely,

James L. Kent

Bibliography and References

Bibliography

Akers B; "The Sacred Mushrooms of Mexico: Assorted Texts". University Press of America, October 10, 2006.

Beyer SV; "Singing to the Plants: A Guide to Mestizo Shamanism in the Upper Amazon". University of New Mexico Press, October 31, 2009.

Cooper JR, Bloom FE, Roth RH; "The Biochemical Basis of Neuropharmacology". Oxford University Press, NY, 7th ed., 1996.

Grinspoon L, Bakalar JB; "Psychedelic Drugs Reconsidered". The Lindesmith Center, 1997.

Grof S; "LSD Psychotherapy". MAPS, 3rd Edition, 2001.

Hayes C; "Tripping: an anthology of true-life psychedelic adventures". Penguin Compass, New York, 2000.

Hobson JA; "The Dream Drugstore: Chemically Altered States of Consciousness". MIT Press, 2001.

Huxley A; "The Doors of Perception". Harper and Row, 1954

LeDoux J; "The Emotional Brain". Simon & Schuster, NY, 1996.

LeDoux J; "Synaptic Self". Viking Penguin, NY, 2002.

Letcher A; "Shroom: A Cultural History of the Magic Mushroom". Faber, Great Britain, 2006.

Lilly JC.; "Programming and Metaprogramming in the Human Biocomputer". Communication Research Institute, 1968.

McKenna T; "The Invisible Landscape". Harper, San Francisco, 1993.

Mullis K; "Dancing Naked in the Mind Field". Vintage, NY, 2000.

Oroc J; "Tryptamine Palace". Park Street Press, Vermont. 2009.

Rabinow P; "Making PCR: a story of biotechnology". University of Chicago Press, 1996

Ruck C, Hofmann A, Wasson GR, et al.; "The Road To Eleusis: Unveiling the Secret of the Mysteries". William Dailey Antiquarian Books, 2004.

Russell D; "Drug War: Covert Money, Power & Policy". Dan Russell, 1999-2000.

Schultes RE, Hofmann A; "Plants of the Gods". Healing Arts Press, Vermont, 1992.

Sheldrake R; "A New Science of Life: The Hypothesis of Morphic Resonance". Park Street Press, Vermont. 1995.

Shulgin A; "TiHKAL: The Continuation". Transform Press, Berkeley, 1997.

Shulgin A; "PiHKAL: A Chemical Love Story". Transform Press, Berkeley, 1991.

Snyder S; "Drugs and The Brain". Scientific American Books, 1986.

Stafford P; "Psychedelics Encyclopedia". Ronin Publishing, Third Edition. 1992.

Stevens J; "Storming Heaven: LSD and the American Dream". Grove Press, 1998.

Stolaraff M; "The Secret Chief: Conversations With a Pioneer of the Underground Psychedelic Therapy Movement ". MAPS, October 1997.

Strassman R; "DMT: The Spirit Molecule". Park Street Press, Vermont. 2001.

Strogatz SH; "Nonlinear Dynamics and Chaos". Perseus Publishing, Cambridge MA, 1994.

Tindall R; "The Jaguar That Roams the Mind". Park Street Press, Vermont, 2008.

Wolfe T; "The Electric Kool-Aid Acid Test". Bantam, 1999.

Zoe 7; "Into The Void". Worldwide Media, 2001.

References

Abraham HD, Duffy FH; "EEG coherence in post-LSD visual hallucinations". Psychiatry Res. 2001 Oct 1;107(3):151-63.

Aghajanian GK, Marek GJ; "Serotonin Induces Excitatory Postsynaptic Potentials in Apical Dendrites of Neocortical Pyramidal Cells". Neuropharmacology Volume 36, Issues 4-5, 5 April 1997, Pages 589-599

Aghajanian GK, Marek GJ; "Seratonin and Hallucinogens". Neuropsychopharmacology. 1999 Aug;21(2 Suppl):16S-23S.

Aghajanian GK, Marek GJ; "Serotonin, via 5-HT2A receptors, increases EPSCs in layer V pyramidal cells of prefrontal cortex by an asynchronous mode of glutamate release". Brain Research 825, Issues 1-2, 17 April 1999, 161-171.

Arnett AM; "Jimson Weed (Datura stramonium) Poisoning". Clinical Toxicology Review Dec 1995, Vol 18 (No 3).

Azmitia EC; "Serotonin and brain: evolution, neuroplasticity, and homeostasis". Int Rev Neurobiol. 2007;77:31-56.

Bach M; "Wagon-wheel effect". From Michael's Optical Illusions & Visual Phenomena. Internet Reference, 2010.

Beer AL, Heckel AH, Greenlee MW; "A Motion Illusion Reveals Mechanisms of Perceptual Stabilization". PLoS ONE 3(7): e2741. 2008.

Behrendt RP; "Hallucinations: synchronisation of thalamocortical gamma oscillations underconstrained by sensory input". Conscious Cogn. 2003 Sep;12(3):413-51.

Belcheva MM, et al.; "μ and κ Opioid Receptors Activate ERK/MAPK via Different Protein Kinase C Isoforms and Secondary Messengers in Astrocytes". J Biol Chem. 2005 July 29; 280(30): 27662–27669.

Bennett-Clarke CA, Chiaia NL, Rhoades RW; "Thalamocortical afferents in rat transiently express high-affinity serotonin uptake sites". Brain Research Volume 733, Issue 2, 16 September 1996, Pages 301-306.

Bohn LM; "Mitogenic Signaling via Endogenous κ-Opioid Receptors in C6 Glioma Cells: Evidence for the Involvement of Protein Kinase C and the Mitogen-Activated Protein Kinase Signaling Cascade". J Neurochem. 2000 February; 74(2): 564–573.

Bokkon I, Kirby M, D'Angiulli A; "TMS, phosphenes and visual mental imagery: A mini-review and a theoretical framework". Symposium on Transcranial Magnetic Stimulation and Neuroimaging in Cognition and Behaviour Conference, Montreal, Quebec, Canada, 25 September 2008.

Bonta IL; "Schizophrenia, dissociative anaesthesia and near-death experience; three events meeting at the NMDA receptor". Med Hypotheses. 2004;62(1).

Boveroux P, et al.; "Brain function in physiologically, pharmacologically, and pathologically altered states of consciousness". Int Anesthesiol Clin. 2008 Summer;46(3):131-46.

Bressloff PC, et al.; "Geometric visual hallucinations, Euclidean symmetry and the functional architecture of striate cortex". Philos Trans R Soc Lond B Biol Sci. 2001 Mar 29;356(1407):299-330.

Bressloff PC, Cowan, et al.; "What Geometric Visual Hallucinations Tell Us about the Visual Cortex". Neural Computation 14 (2002) 473–491.

Brown University; "Scientists explain inception of perception in the brain". Physorg, March 5, 2007.

Bruchas MR, et al.; "Kappa Opioid Receptor Activation of p38 MAPK Is GRK3- and Arrestin-dependent in Neurons and Astrocytes". June 30, 2006 The Journal of Biological Chemistry, 281, 18081-18089.

Buckman, J; "Brainwashing, LSD, and CIA: Historical and Ethical Perspective". International Journal of Social Psychiatry, Vol. 23, No. 1, 8-19 (1977).

Burnet PW, Eastwood SL, et al.; "The distribution of 5-HT1A and 5-HT2A receptor mRNA in human brain". Brain Res. 1995 Apr 3;676(1):157-68.

Busch N, Dubois J, VanRullen R; "The Phase of Ongoing EEG Oscillations Predicts Visual Perception". The Journal of Neuroscience, June 17, 2009, 29(24):7869-7876.

Butters, Nelson; "The effect of LSD-25 on spatial and stimulus perseverative tendencies in rats". Psychopharmacology 8:6, November, 1966.

Cerrito E, et al.; "5HT2-receptors and serotonin release: Their role in human platelet aggregation". Life Sciences Volume 53, Issue 3, 1993, 209-215.

Charing HG; "Communion with the Infinite: The visual music of the Shipibo people of the Amazon". SH, Winter 2005.

Chizhevsky VN, Corbalan R; "Multistability in a driven nonlinear system controlled by weak subharmonic perturbations". phycon, vol. 2, pp.396-402, 2003 International Conference on Physics and Control.

Cho RY, Konecky RO, Carter CS; "Impairments in frontal cortical gamma synchrony and cognitive control in schizophrenia". Proc Natl Acad Sci U S A. 2006 Dec 26;103(52):19878-83.

Christiansen A, Baum R, Witt P; "Changes In Spider Webs Brought About By Mescaline, Psilocybin And An Increase In Body Weight". JPET April 1962 vol.136 no.1 31-37.

Cochen V, Arnulf I, Demeret S, et al.; "Vivid dreams, hallucinations, psychosis and REM sleep in Guillain-Barré syndrome". Brain, ISSN 0006-8950. 2005, vol. 128 (11), pp. 2535-2545.

Colgin, Laura Lee, et al.; "Frequency of gamma oscillations routes flow of information in the hippocampus". Nature 462, 353-357 (19 November 2009).

Connely B; "Neuropharmacology of Hallucinogens : a brief introduction". Erowid.org, Internet Reference, 2004.

Connors C; "Bypassing interneurons: inhibition in neocortex". Nature Neuroscience 10, 808 - 810 (2007).

Coren, S; "Sleep Deprivation, Psychosis and Mental Efficiency". Psychiatric Times. Vol. 15 No. 3, 1998.

Corlett PR, Frith CD, Fletcher PC; "From drugs to deprivation: a Bayesian framework for understanding models of psychosis". Psychopharmacology (Berl). 2009 November; 206(4): 515–530.

Davis M, Walters JK; "Psilocybin: biphasic dose-response effects on the acoustic startle reflex in the rat". Pharmacol Biochem Behav. 1977 Apr;6(4):427-31.

Deering MF; "Limits of Human Vision". Sun Microsystems Internal, 1998.

Deschenes M, Bourassa J, Pinault, D ; "Corticothalamic projections from layer V cells in rat are collaterals of long-range corticofugal axons". Brain-Res. 1994 Nov 21; 664(1-2): 215-9

Dobelle WH, Mladejovsky HG; "Phosphenes produced by electrical stimulation of human occipital cortex, and their application to the development of a prosthesis for the blind". J Physiol. 1974 December; 243(2): 553–576.1.

Doblin, R; "Pahnke's "Good Friday Experiment' A Long-Term Follow-Up And Methodological Critique". The Journal of Transpersonal Psychology, Vol. 23, No. 1, 1991.

Douglas, Koch, Mahowald, Martin, Suarez; "Recurrent Excitation in Neocortical Circuits". Science 269-5226 (1995) 981-985.

Eagleman D, Pariyadath V; "Is subjective duration a signature of coding efficiency?". Phil. Trans. R. Soc. B 12 July 2009 vol. 364 no. 1525 1841-1851.

Ermentrout B; "Dynamical consequences of fast-rising, slow-decaying synapses in neuronal networks". Neural Computation 15-11 (2003) 2483 - 2522.

Ermentrout, Cowen; "A mathematical theory of visual hallucination patterns". Biological Cybernetics 34-3 (1979) 137-150.

Erowid.org; "Erowid Experience Vaults". Internet Reference, 2010.

Erowid.org; "Peyote Legal Status". Internet Reference, 2010.

Erowid.org; "UDV Wins Supreme Court Decision on Preliminary Injunction Allowing the use of their ayahuasca / hoasca tea". Internet Reference, 2010.

Fischer R, Hill R, Thatcher K, Scheib J.; "Psilocybin-induced contraction of nearby visual space". Agents Actions. 1970 Aug;1(4):190-7.

Fischer R, Hill RM, Warshay D; "Effects of psychodysleptic drug psilocybin on visual perception. Changes in brightness preference". Experientia. 1969 Feb 15;25(2):166-9.

Forutan F, Estalji S, Beu M, et al.; "Distribution of 5HT2A receptors in the human brain: comparison of data in vivo and post mortem". Nuklearmedizin. 2002;41(4):197-201.

Fox D; "Timewarp: How your brain creates the fourth dimension". New Scientist, Issue 2731, 21 October 2009.

Gao, Krimer, Goldman-Rakic; "Presynaptic regulation of recurrent excitation by D1 receptors in prefrontal circuits". PNAS 98-1, 295-300, 2001.

Geyer MA, Vollenweider FX; "Serotonin research: contributions to understanding psychoses". Trends Pharmacol Sci. 2008 Sep;29(9):445-53.

Glennon RA, et al.; "Evidence for 5-HT2 involvement in the mechanism of action of hallucinogenic agents". Life Sci. 1984 Dec 17;35(25):2505-11.

Gokalp, G; "Sleep and Dreams". Internet Reference, 1999

Gresch PJ, et al.; "Behavioral tolerance to lysergic acid diethylamide is associated with reduced serotonin-2A receptor signaling in rat cortex". Neuropsychopharmacology. 2005 Sep;30(9):1693-702.

Griffiths RR, Richards WA, et al.; "Mystical-type experiences occasioned by psilocybin mediate the attribution of personal meaning and spiritual significance 14 months later". Journal of Psychopharmacology, Vol. 22, No. 6, 621-632 (2008).

Griffiths RR; "Psilocybin can occasion mystical-type experiences having substantial and sustained personal meaning and spiritual significance". Psychopharmacology (2006) 187:268–283.

Gutkin, Pinto, Ermentrout; "Mathematical Neuroscience: From Neurons to Circuits to Systems". Journal of Physiology - Paris 97 (2003) 209–219.

Harner MJ; "Common Themes in South American Indian Yage Experiences". Internet Reference, 2010.

Hasler F, Grimberg U, Benz M, Huber T, Vollenweider F; "Acute psychological and physiological effects of psilocybin in healthy humans: a double-blind, placebo-controlled dose-effect study". Psychopharmacology, Volume 172, Number 2 / March, 2004

HHS/SAMHSA, Office of Applied Studies; "Ecstasy, Other Club Drugs, & Other Hallucinogens". Internet Reference, 2008.

Hill RM, Fischer R; "Interpretation of visual space under drug-induced ergotropic and trophotropic arousal". Agents Actions. 1971 Nov;2(3):122-30.

Hobson JA, Stickgold R, Pace-Schott EF; "The neuropsychology of REM sleep dreaming". NeuroReport: 16 February 1998 - Volume 9 - Issue 3 - p R1-R14.

Hoffmann E; "Effects of a Psychedelic, Tropical Tea, Ayahuasca, on the Electroencephalographic (EEG) Activity of the Human Brain during a Shamanistic Ritual". MAPS Spring (2001) 25-30.

Itil TM; "Anticholinergic drug-induced sleep-like EEG pattern in man". Psychopharmacologia. 1969;14(5):383-93.

Jakab RL, Goldman-Rakic PS; "5-Hydroxytryptamine2A serotonin receptors in the primate cerebral cortex: Possible site of action of hallucinogenic and antipsychotic drugs in pyramidal cell apical dendrites". PNAS January 20, 1998 vol. 95 no. 2 735-740.

Jarvik M, Chorover S; "Impairment by lysergic acid diethylamide of accuracy in performance of a delayed alternation test in monkeys". Psychopharmacology, Volume 1, Number 3 / May, 1960.

Jones EG; "Thalamic circuitry and thalamocortical synchrony". Philos Trans R Soc Lond B Biol Sci. 2002 Dec 29;357(1428):1659-73.

Judd LL, McAdams L, Budnick B, Braff DL ; "Sensory gating deficits in schizophrenia: new results". Am J Psychiatry 1992; 149:488-493.

Kanamaru, T., "Van der Pol oscillator", *Scholarpedia*, 2(1), 2202, (2007).

Kass L, Hartline PH, Adolph AR ; "Presynaptic uptake blockade hypothesis for LSD action at the lateral inhibitory synapse in Limulus". The Journal of General Physiology, Vol 82, 245-267.

Kent JL; "Psychedelic Information Theory: Alpha Edition". Tripzine.com, Internet Reference, 2004.

Kent JL; "Signal Theory Overview". Tripzine.com, Internet Reference, 2006.

Kent JL; "Signal Theory Poster". Towards a Science of Consciousness Conference, Tucson, AZ, 2006.

Kent JL; "Selective 5-HT2A agonist hallucinogens: A review of pharmacological interaction and corollary perceptual effects". Tripzine.com, Internet Reference, 2008.

Kent JL, Pickover C; "The Case Against DMT Elves". Tripzine.com, Internet Reference, 2004.

Kittenis M., Caryl PG, Stevens P; "Distant psychophysiological interaction effects between related and unrelated participants". Association 47th Annual Convention: Proceedings of Presented Papers, Vienna (67-76), 2004.

Knoll M, Kuglerb J, et al.; "Effects of Chemical Stimulation of Electrically-Induced Phosphenes on their Bandwidth, Shape, Number and Intensity". Sterotactic and Functional Neurosurgery, Vol. 23, No. 3, 1963.

Levitated.net; "Artifacts of Computation". Internet Reference.

Lehar, S; "Harmonic Resonance in the Brain: Spatial patterns in perception and behavior mediated by spatial standing waves in neural tissue". Internet Reference, 2010.

Luke D; "Psi-verts and Psychic Piracy: The Future of Parapsychology?". Reality Sandwich, Internet Reference, 7-6-09.

Lumer ED, Edelman GM, Tononi G; "Neural dynamics in a model of the thalamocortical system. II. The role of neural synchrony tested through perturbations of spike timing". Cereb Cortex. 1997 Apr-May;7(3):228-36.

Marc Wittmann, et al; "Effects of psilocybin on time perception and temporal control of behaviour in humans". 2007;21:50.

Mason OJ, Brady F; "The psychotomimetic effects of short-term sensory deprivation". J Nerv Ment Dis. 2009 Oct;197(10):783-5.

McLean TH, Parrish JC, Braden MR, Marona-Lewicka D, Gallardo-Godoy A, Nichols DE; "1-Aminomethylbenzocycloalkanes: conformationally-restricted hallucinogenic phenethylamine analogues as functionally-selective 5 HT2A receptor agonists". J Med Chem. 2006 Sep 21;49(19):5794-803.

Meador KJ, et al.; "Gamma coherence and conscious perception". Neurology 2002;59:847-854.

Melechi A, "Seeing Stars: The Shifting Geometry of Phosphenes". Trip Magazine, issue 10, 26-27, 2004.

Meredith MA, Stein BE; "Visual, auditory, and somatosensory convergence on cells in superior colliculus results in multisensory integration". J Neurophysiol 56: 640-662, 1986.

Miller RE, Tredici TJ; "Vision Manual for the Flight Surgeon: The Eye and Night Vision". USAF Special Report, AL-SR-1992-0002.

Mishlove J; "Interview with Francis Crick". Transcript from 'Thinking Allowed, Conversations On the Leading Edge of Knowledge and Discovery'.

Munglani R, Jones JG; "Sleep and General Anesthesia as Altered States of Consciousness". Journal of Psychopharmacology 6:399-409, 1992.

Nichols CD, Sanders-Bush E; "A Single Dose of Lysergic Acid Diethylamide Influences Gene Expression Patterns within the Mammalian Brain". Neuropsychopharmacology (2002) 26 634-642.

Nichols DE; "Hallucinogens". Pharmacology & Therapeutics Volume 101, Issue 2, February 2004, Pages 131-181.

Nicholson PT, Firnhaber RP; "Autohypnotic Induction of Sleep Rhythms Generates Visions of Light with Form-constant Patterns". White Paper.

Norwegian University of Science and Technology (NTNU); "How the Brain Filters out Distracting Thoughts to Focus on a Single Bit of Information". ScienceDaily 23 November 2009.

Pantone, DJ; "The Shipibo Indians: Masters of Ayahuasca". Internet Reference, 2006.

Payne JD, Nadel L.; "Sleep, dreams, and memory consolidation: the role of the stress hormone cortisol". Learn Mem. 2004 Nov-Dec;11(6):671-8.

Pettifor E; "Altered States: The Origin of Art in Entoptic Phenomena". Internet Reference, 1996.

Pickover C; "DMT, Moses, and the Quest for Transcendence". Reality Carnival, 'Sex, Drugs, Einstein, and Elves', 2004.

Pinto B, Ermentrout B; "Spatially Structured Activity In Synaptically Coupled Neuronal Networks: I. Traveling Fronts And Pulses". SIAM J. Appl. Math 62-1 (2001) 226-243.

Pompeiano M, Palacios JM, Mengod G.; "Distribution of the serotonin 5-HT2 receptor family mRNAs: comparison between 5-HT2A and 5-HT2C receptors". Brain Res Mol Brain Res. 1994 Apr;23(1-2):163-78.

Prudence, Paul; "Chaotic fingerprints and space-time labyrinths". Internet Reference, 2005.

Pöppel E; "Pre-semantically defined temporal windows for cognitive processing". Phil. Trans. R. Soc. B 12 July 2009 vol. 364 no. 1525 1887-1896.

Rampe J; "Softology - Video Feedback". Internet Reference.

Ray TS; "Psychedelics and the Human Receptorome". PLoS One. 2010; 5(2): e9019.

Rees, Alun; "Nobel Prize genius Crick was high on LSD when he discovered the secret of life". Mail on Sunday, 8 August 2004.

Riba J, Anderer P, et al.; "Topographic pharmaco-EEG mapping of the effects of the South American psychoactive beverage ayahuasca in healthy volunteers". Br J Clin Pharmacol. 2002 June; 53(6): 613–628.

Riba J, Anderer P, et al.; "Effects of the South American Psychoactive Beverage Ayahuasca on Regional Brain Electrical Activity in Humans: A Functional Neuroimaging Study". Neuropsychobiology 2004;50:89-101.

Richards TL, Kozak et al.; "Replicable functional magnetic resonance imaging evidence of correlated brain signals between physically isolated subjects.". Journal of Alternative and Complementary Medicine, 11, 955-963.

Rose D, Horn G; "Effects of LSD on the responses of single units in cat visual cortex". Experimental Brain Research, Volume 27, Number 1 / January, 1977.

Sabolek HR, Penley SC, et al.; "Theta and gamma coherence along the septotemporal axis of the hippocampus". J Neurophysiol. 2009 Mar;101(3):1192-200.

Sadzot B, Baraban JM, et al.; "Hallucinogenic drug interactions at human brain 5-HT2 receptors: implications for treating LSD-induced hallucinogenesis". Psychopharmacology (Berl). 1989;98(4):495-9.

Sattelkau T; "An Interview with Dave Nichols". Trip Magazine, Vol 5., Spring 2000, p 42.

Scienceblog.com; "Does time dilate during a threatening situation?". Internet Reference, January 23, 2010.

Shao Z, Burkhalter A; "Role of GABAB receptor-mediated inhibition in reciprocal interareal pathways of rat visual cortex". J Neurophysiol. 1999 Mar;81(3):1014-24.

Shema R, Sacktor TC, Dudai Y; "Rapid erasure of long-term memory associations in the cortex by an inhibitor of PKM zeta". Science. 2007 Aug 17;317(5840):951-3.

Siegel JM; "The stuff dreams are made of: anatomical substrates of REM sleep". Nature Neuroscience, V9.6, p721, 06/2006.

Sipes TE, Geyer MA; "DOI disrupts prepulse inhibition of startle in rats via 5-HT2A receptors in the ventral pallidum.". Brain Res. 1997 Jun 27;761(1):97-104.

Spratling MW; "Cortical Region Interactions and the Functional Role of Apical Dendrites". Behavioral and Cognitive Neuroscience 1-3 (2002) 219-228.

Stickgold R, Hobson JA, Fosse R, Fosse M; "Sleep, learning, and dreams: off-line memory reprocessing". Science. 2001 Nov 2;294(5544):1052-7.

Stuckey DE, Lawson R, Luna LE; "EEG gamma coherence and other correlates of subjective reports during ayahuasca experiences". J Psychoactive Drugs. 2005 Jun;37(2):163-78.

Swaminathan, Nikhil; "How Hallucinogens Play Their Mind-Bending Games". Scientific American, January 31, 2007.

Taylor RP, Sprott JC.; "Biophilic fractals and the visual journey of organic screen-savers". Nonlinear Dynamics Psychol Life Sci. 2008 Jan;12(1):117-29.

Trulson M, Howell G; "Ontogeny of the behavioral effects of lysergic acid diethylamide in cats". Developmental Psychobiology 17:4, 329 – 346.

Urban JD, et al.; "Functional selectivity and classical concepts of quantitative pharmacology". J Pharmacol Exp Ther. 2007 Jan;320(1):1-13.

VanRullen R, Pascual-Leone A, Battelli L; "The Continuous Wagon Wheel Illusion and the "When' Pathway of the Right Parietal Lobe: A Repetitive Transcranial Magnetic Stimulation Study". PLoS ONE 3(8): e2911. August 6, 2008.

VanRullen R, et al.; "The continuous Wagon Wheel Illusion is object-based". Vision Research Volume 46, Issue 24, November 2006, Pages 4091-4095.

Vollenweider FX, Geyer MA; "A systems model of altered consciousness: integrating natural and drug-induced psychoses". Brain Res Bull. 2001 Nov 15;56(5):495-507.

Wasson RG; "Seeking the Magic Mushroom". Life Magazine, May 13, 1957, p100.

Watts SW; "Activation of the mitogen-activated protein kinase pathway via the 5-HT2A receptor". Ann N Y Acad Sci. 1998 Dec 15;861:162-8.

WikiPedia.org; "Interference (wave propagation)". Internet Reference, 2010.

WikiPedia.org; "Chaos Magic". Internet Reference, 2010.

WikiPedia.org; "Mitogen-activated protein kinase". Internet Reference, 2010.

WikiPedia.org; "Space-filling Curves". Internet Reference, 2010.

WikiPedia.org; "5-HT2A Receptor". Internet Reference, 2010.

WikiPedia.org; "Protein kinase C". Internet Reference, 2010.

WikiPedia.org; "Nonlinear System". Internet Reference, 2010.

WikiPedia.org; "Stockholm Syndrome". Internet Reference, 2010.

WikiPedia.org; "Distributed Cognition". Internet Reference, 2010.

WikiPedia.org; "Electroencephalography". Internet Reference, 2010.

WikiPedia.org; "Subliminal stimuli". Internet Reference, 2010.

WikiPedia.org; "Wagon wheel effect". Internet Reference, 2010.

WikiPedia.org; "Working memory". Internet Reference, 2010.

WikiPedia.org; "Retina". Internet Reference, 2010.

WikiPedia.org; "Grid illusion". Internet Reference, 2010.

WikiPedia.org; "Kalachakra". Internet Reference, 2010.

WikiPedia.org; "Watchmaker analogy". Internet Reference, 2010.

WikiPedia.org; "Hermeticism". Internet Reference, 2010.

WikiPedia.org; "Visible spectrum". Internet Reference, 2010.

WikiPedia.org; "Control Theory". Internet Reference, 2010.

WikiPedia.org; "Entrainment (Physics)". Internet Reference, 2009.

WikiPedia.org; "ADSR envelope". Internet Reference, 2009.

WikiPedia.org; "Symbionese Liberation Army". Internet Reference, 2010.

WikiPedia.org; "Aum Shinrikyo". Internet Reference, 2010.

WikiPedia.org; "Project MKULTRA". Internet Reference, 2010.

WikiPedia.org; "Peripheral drift illusion". Internet Reference, 2008.

Williams JD, Dowson TA, et al. ; "The Signs of All Times: Entoptic Phenomena in Upper Palaeolithic Art". Current Anthropology, Vol. 29, No. 2 (Apr., 1988), pp. 201-245 .

Wolfram Math; "Peano Curves". Internet Reference, 2010.

Wolfram Math; "Hilbert and Moore Fractal Curves". Internet Reference, 2010.

Wolfram Math; "Wunderlich Curves". Internet Reference, 2010.

Yu B, et al.; "Serotonin 5-Hydroxytryptamine2A Receptor Activation Suppresses Tumor Necrosis Factor-α-Induced Inflammation with Extraordinary Potency". JPET November 2008 vol. 327 no. 2 316-323.

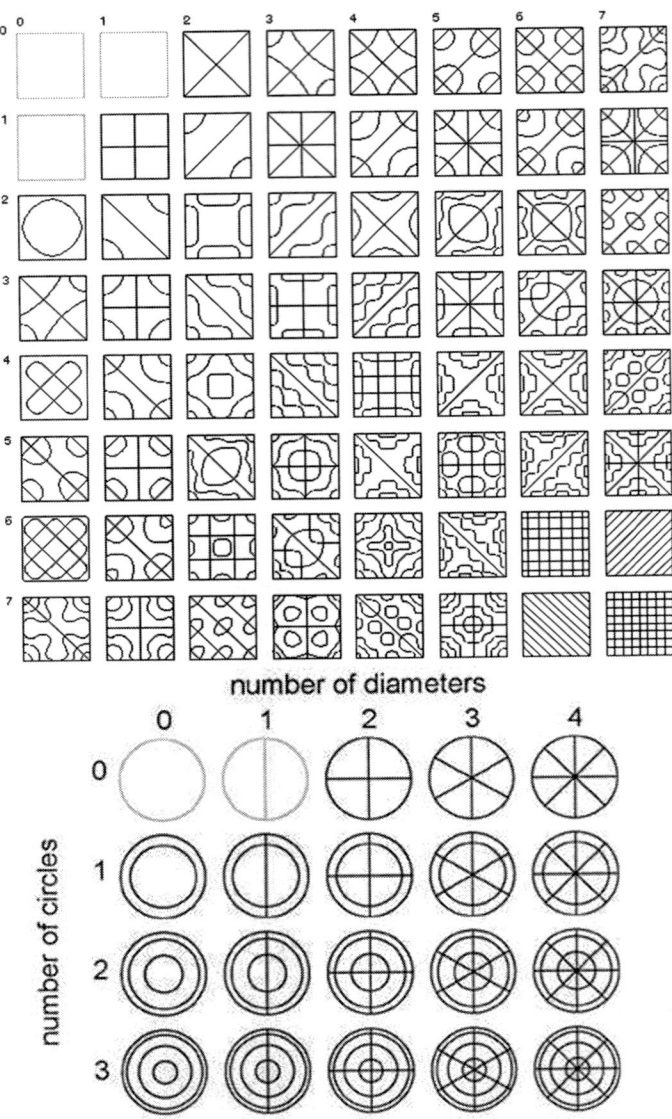

Figure 31. Chladni figures for a square steel plate (top) and a circular plate (bottom) demonstrate the variety of standing wave patterns generated in simple resonating systems. Examining the physical properties of standing waves in resonant systems is also called cymatics. Archetypal forms generated in both rectangular and circular plates are isomorphic of flicker phosphenes seen at various frequencies of light pulse stimulation, and have been reproduced in textile patterns, ceramics, and sacred mandalas since roughly 10,000 BCE. From Lehar, 2010.

About the Author

James L. Kent is a writer and programmer living in Seattle, Washington, and has studied hallucinogens and perception for over twenty years. He is the former Editor of *Psychedelic Illuminations Magazine*, the former Publisher of *Trip Magazine: The Journal of Psychedelic Culture*. and the creator and co-editor of *DoseNation.com*, a web log for drug news, media, culture, and humor. He is also a contributing neuroscience columnist for *h+ Magazine*.

LaVergne, TN USA
20 March 2011
220884LV00004B/144/P